DISORDERS
of the
HORSE

Their Cause, Symptoms & Treatment

BY ELSIE HANAUER

Published by
Melvin Powers
WILSHIRE BOOK COMPANY
12015 Sherman Road
No. Hollywood, California 91605
Telephone: (213) 875-1711

Library of Congress Cataloging in Publication Data

Hanauer, Elsie V
    Disorders of the horse.

    Bibliography: p.
    1. Horses—Diseases.   I. Title.
SF951.H23   636.1′08′9   72-6364
ISBN 0-498-01256-5

To Geri Lu, Barbie & Trudy,
my friends and fellow horsemen

Printed by

HAL LEIGHTON PRINTING COMPANY
P.O. Box 3952
North Hollywood, California 91605
Telephone: (213) 983-1105

ISBN 0-87980-281-2
PRINTED IN THE UNITED STATES OF AMERICA

Contents

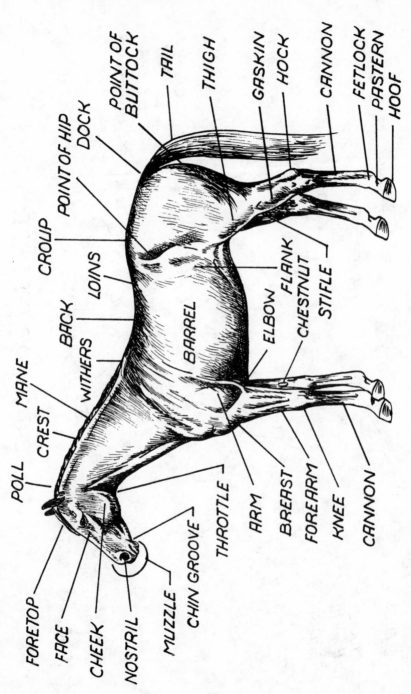

POINTS OF THE HORSE

POLL
MANE
CREST
FORETOP
FACE
CHEEK
NOSTRIL
MUZZLE
CHIN GROOVE
THROTTLE
ARM
BREAST
FOREARM
KNEE
CANNON
WITHERS
BACK
LOINS
CROUP
POINT OF HIP
DOCK
POINT OF BUTTOCK
TAIL
THIGH
GASKIN
HOCK
CANNON
FETLOCK
PASTERN
HOOF
BARREL
ELBOW
FLANK
CHESTNUT
STIFLE

11

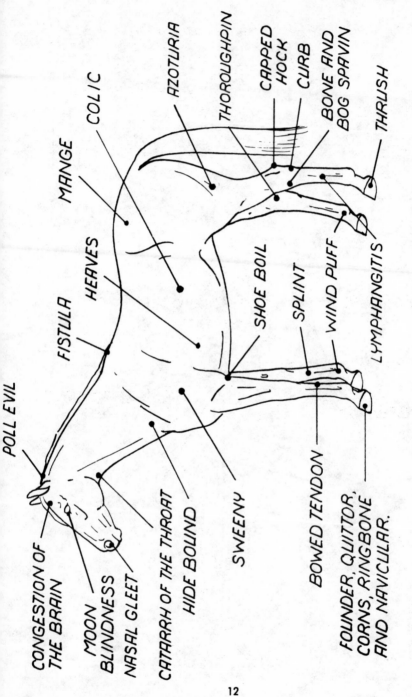

LOCATION OF DISORDERS

POLL EVIL
CONGESTION OF THE BRAIN
MOON BLINDNESS
NASAL GLEET
CATARRH OF THE THROAT
HIDE BOUND
SWEENY
BOWED TENDON
FOUNDER, QUITTOR, CORNS, RINGBONE AND NAVICULAR.
LYMPHANGITIS
WIND PUFF
SPLINT
SHOE BOIL
FISTULA
HEAVES
MANGE
COLIC
AZOTURIA
THOROUGHPIN
CAPPED HOCK
CURB
BONE AND BOG SPAVIN
THRUSH

12

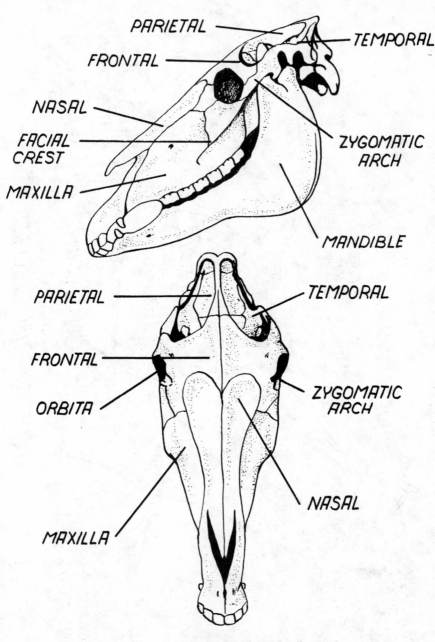

PARIETAL

TEMPORAL

FRONTAL

NASAL

FACIAL
CREST

MAXILLA

ZYGOMATIC
ARCH

MANDIBLE

PARIETAL

TEMPORAL

FRONTAL

ORBITA

ZYGOMATIC
ARCH

NASAL

MAXILLA

THE SKULL

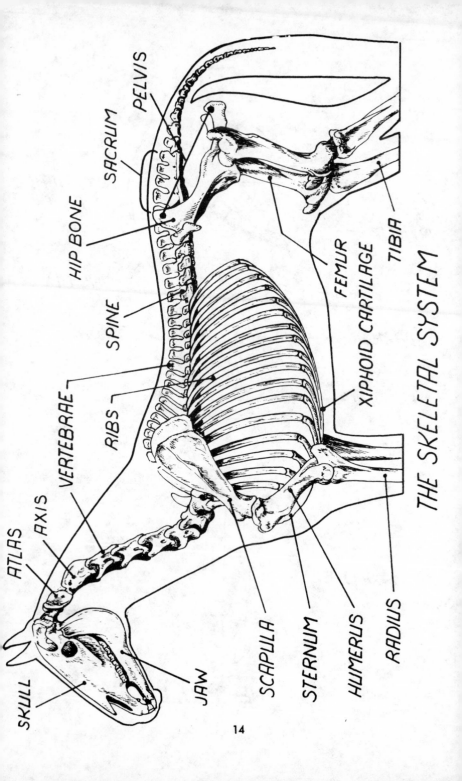

THE SKELETAL SYSTEM

ATLAS
AXIS
SKULL
JAW
SCAPULA
STERNUM
HUMERUS
RADIUS
VERTEBRAE
RIBS
SPINE
HIP BONE
SACRUM
PELVIS
FEMUR
XIPHOID CARTILAGE
TIBIA

14

Diagnosis

Diagnosis, History, Attitude, The Skin, Visible Mucous Membranes, Respirations, Appetite And Thirst, The Urine, The Pulse, The Temperature, Fever.

QUIET ATTITUDE.

SWEATING.

DULL COAT.

LABOURED BREATHING.

SKIN ERUPTIONS.

CONSTIPATION.

DROOPING HEAD AND NECK.

DIARRHEA.

ABDOMINAL SWELLING.

RESTING OF FEET ALTERNATELY.

COUGH

NASAL DISCHARGE.

ANXIOUS OR HAGGERED EXPRESSION.

POOR APPETITE.

INDICATIONS OF DISORDER

16

Diagnosis

When examining a horse to diagnosis a disorder, a thorough knowledge of the conditions that exist in health is highly important because it is by the knowledge of what is normal that one is generally able to detect abnormal conditions. It should be remembered when trying to make a diagnosis that symptoms of disorders are not always evident and few are peculiar to any particular disease. Complications often obscure the original affliction. It should be remembered, too, that horses of different breeds or families often act differently under the influence of the same disorder. Hence a degree of fever that does not produce marked dullness in one horse may cause the most serious dejection in another horse.

History

It is always important to know something of the origin and development of a disorder. The cause of a disorder is important for diagnosis and proper treatment. The food the horse has eaten, the type of work he has done, the care he has received, and the places he has been should all be carefuly investigated.

Attitude

Special attention should always be paid to the horse's attitude. Often horses will assume positions that are characteristic of a certain disorder. For example, a horse with colic may sit upon his haunches or balance himself upon his back. A sick horse who refuses to lie down may have a respiratory disorder. Frequent lying down or lying down at unusual times or places is generally an indication of a disorder. Depressed head, drooping ears, feet rested alternately, an anxious or haggard expression, and dullness all generally indicate disorder.

The Skin

The condition of the skin is generally a good indication of a horse's physical condition, as there is no part of the body that loses its tone and elasticity as a result of disease quicker than the skin. The horse's coat, normally fine, smooth, and glossy, is in disease generally dry, lusterless, and staring. Delay in changing the coat, loss of hair, scaliness, and any thickening, swelling, or eruptions of the skin are indications of disorder.

Extreme warmth of the skin is usually present in high fevers. Horses often sweat freely when there is a serious respiratory disorder or very intense pain. Local sweating (sweating of a restricted area) often denotes some kind of nerve interference. Cold, clammy sweating is frequently seen in disorders which cause considerable pain.

Visible Mucous Membranes

The condition of a horse is often reflected to a certain extent by the appearance of the mucous membranes. Any change in these membranes can be easily seen in the lining of the eyelids or in the lining of the nostrils. Normally the membranes are a slightly pink color, thus paleness or redness indicate disorder. Fever and pain often cause increased redness. Serious disorders of the heart or respiratory system may cause the membranes to become a bluish color, while a liver condition generally causes them to become yellowish.

Respiration

Respirations may be noted over the flank or at the nostrils. The normal rate of respirations for a healthy horse at rest is 8–16 times per minute, the rate being much faster in young animals than in old. Respirations can be counted for 30 seconds and then calculated for one minute. Acceleration of the respiratory rate may be caused by fever, lung disorders, pain, and constriction of the air passages leading to the lungs. In labored or difficult respiration, the horse will often stand with his front feet apart, the neck straight out, and the head extended. The nostrils are generally widely dilated and the face may show an anxious expression.

Appetite and Thirst

A healthy horse normally has a good appetite, but fever, digestive disturbances, bad or sharp teeth, and pain generally cause a loss of appetite. The desire to eat abnormal things such as dirty bedding, manure, rotten wood, or soil is often caused by indigestion, worms, or a mineral deficiency. An abnormal thirst is often present with fever, diarrhea, or diabetes. A lack of desire for water is common in colic and many disorders of an acute nature.

The Urine

The urine is a frequent indicator of disorder. The amount will generally vary with weather, exercise, and the type of food and water taken in. Normal urination occurs about six to eleven times a day. The urine of a healthy horse is nearly always turbid (more so in some horses than others). The normal color is yellow or yellowish red, and the color is less intense when the quantity is large. Frequent attempts to urinate, painful urination, reddish or brownish urine, urine passed in drops or in a small stream, and passage of blood in the urine are all indications of disorder.

The Pulse

The pulse or heart rate is normally accelerated by digestion of food, hot weather, exercise, and excitement. In health the pulse is regular, separate beats of equal fullness or volume following each other after intervals of equal length. The normal pulse rate in a healthy horse at rest is 36–40 beats per minute. It should be remembered that the rate is normally much faster in young horses than in mature ones: for example, a foal two to four weeks old may have a pulse of 80–100 beats per minute.

Disorders may cause the pulse to become slower or faster than normal. Slowing of the pulse may be caused by exhaustion, excessive cold, old age, and certain drugs. A rapid pulse is generally found in fevers. The more severe the infection and the weaker the heart, the more rapid the pulse: in heart disorders the pulse is generally very rapid. When the pulse rate rises above 100 beats per minute, recovery is not promising.

The pulse of a horse may be taken at any point where a large artery is close to the skin and above a bone, cartilage, or tendon. The most convenient place for taking the pulse is at the jaw in front of the heavy cheek muscles, where the maxillary artery runs from between the jaws, around the lower border of the jawbone, and up on the outside of the jawbone. The tips of the fingers should be pressed lightly on the skin over the artery to feel the distinctive throb.

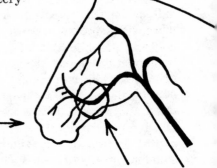

PULSE MAY BE TAKEN IN AREA INDICATED. →

The Temperature

The normal temperature of a horse will vary somewhat under different conditions. It is normally higher in young animals than in older ones, higher in hot weather than in cold, and higher at night than in the morning. The normal temperature of a healthy, mature horse generally varies from 99.5° to 101° Fahrenheit. A temperature of 102.5° is a low fever, 104° a moderate fever, and 106° a high fever. A temperature of 107.5° is considered dangerous. In some disorders the temperature may go as high as 110°, but in infectious diseases it rarely exceeds 106°

The temperature of a horse is generally measured with a veterinarian's rectal thermometer around six inches long. Shake the mercury to 95° and insert the bulb end until three quarters of it is within. Leave it in position for two minutes before withdrawing it.

Fever

In the cold stages of a fever the horse may shiver frequently, the surface of his body may be cold, and respirations generally increase in frequency. The pulse may be low and the mucous membranes dry. The appetite is usually poor, the urine scanty, and evacuation difficult. Constipation may be present.

In the hot stages of a fever the horse generally appears dull, while the respirations and pulse are increased. The mucous membranes are usually red, the extremities may be hot, and the breath is offensive. The manure is noticeably lighter in color and harder than normal. The quantity of urine decreases and it is darker in color. The appetite is lost. The hot stage of a fever generally lasts longer than the cold stage and commonly persists until convalescence or death. If a fever continues for a long period and is associated with a poor or lost appetite, the horse will lose a considerable amount of weight.

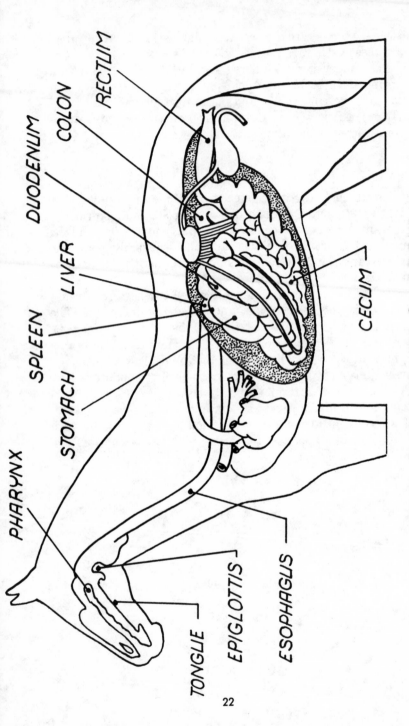

THE DIGESTIVE SYSTEM

22

The Digestive System

Teeth, Choking, Colic, Flatulent Colic, Spasmodic Colic, Impaction Of The Large Intestines, Gastro-Enteritis, Peritonitis, Diarrhea, Defecation, Internal Parasites.

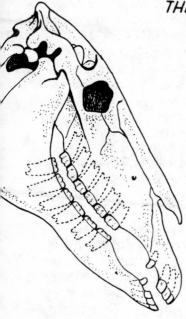

A HORSE SKULL SHOWING POSITION OF TEETH AND THEIR ROOTS.

Teeth

The front teeth of the horse are used for biting and grasping, aiding the lips in bringing food into the mouth. The back teeth grind the food. Thus the teeth are actually the first stage of the digestive system.

Ordinarily a horse's teeth are healthy and free of decay (such as that experienced by humans), but age and wear often lead to sharp molars, which do require attention. The upper jaw of the horse is somewhat wider than the lower, and the fact that the teeth are not perfectly opposed means that sharp ridges are left unworn on the inside of the lower molars and on the outside of the upper molars. These sharp ridges may cut the inside of the cheek, injure the tongue, and prevent the horse from masticating food properly. Sharp molars generally lead to an abundance of saliva and to masses of semi-masticated food being lodged between the teeth and cheeks. The horse may eat very slowly, food may fall from the mouth, and the head is often held to one side while chewing.

Sharp molars are generally corrected by a method known as "floating." A special tooth rasp, placed between the cheek and the upper molars, is carefully moved forward and back, smoothing the outside edges of the upper molars. The lower molars normally do not require floating. This service should be performed by an experienced hand, as an inexperienced person could easily injure the horse's cheek or tongue.

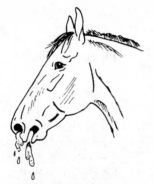

Choking is infrequent in horses. It is generally caused by the animal accidentally swallowing food before it is properly masticated. The appearance of sudden or frightening disturbances while the horse is eating commonly cause choking. Greedy animals who bolt their food are also susceptible to it.

EXCESS SALIVA AND PORTIONS OF FOOD ARE EJECTED FROM THE NOSTRILS AND MOUTH.

Symptoms of choking are generally a sudden difficulty or complete inability to swallow. There is profuse salivation and portions of food may be ejected from the mouth and nostrils. There are repeated retching movements and the horse shows marked evidence of distress. There may be fits of coughing and convulsive trembling of muscles. As these symptoms are often alarming, great discrimination is necessary for the attendant. The inexperienced person must not hastily attempt to remove lodged matter.

When choking is caused by lodged grain, hay, or pellets, it will normally diminish in a short time with the excessive flow of saliva, tending to disappear spontaneously. In these cases it is generally best to turn the horse into a large box stall or corral, removing all food materials and objects that could cause injury. Those cases which have choked on carrots, apples, or other materials which are not easily dissolved, should have immediate attention from a veterinarian. Unless directed by a veterinarian, the inexperienced should not attempt drenching or using a stomach tube. The results could prove fatal.

Once a horse has choked, it is often wise to withhold all food for three or four hours. Then feed the horse a warm bran mash. If the esophagus was badly irritated from the lodged matter, coarse food taken too soon could cause a repeated attack. The bran mash is soothing to irritated tissues.

Colic, a term referring to a group of symptoms which indicate severe abdominal pain, is a common disorder in horses: this can be attributed to the animal's small stomach, his inability to vomit, the great length of the intestines, and the puckering of the large intestine.

The most common causes of colic are irregularity in feeding, sudden changes in diet, withered greens or moldy hay, eating while fatigued, insufficient water, poor mastication of foods, hard work immediately after eating, and parasites. It is plain to see from this that in most instances the owner is at fault; most cases of colic can be avoided through proper care.

Colic is generally characterized by severe abdominal pain. This pain is clearly indicated by the horse's considerable restlessness, pawing, looking at the flanks, yawning, lying down, rolling, frequent changes in position, and groaning. In severe colic attacks the horse may run in delirium or throw himself to the ground, kicking and rolling violently. Breathing may be labored and the body may become drenched with sweat.

At the first indications of colic, withhold all food and summon a veterinarian. Walk the horse quietly if desired, but never force him to trot or run, or allow violent rolling. These actions could result in the rupture of an organ. Hot towels or blankets applied to the belly and flanks will help reduce pain and stimulate bowel action. Drenches or any other suggested concoctions should be avoided, as improper treatment can do harm.

Horses recovering from colic should not be fed a full ration for 24 to 48 hours, depending upon the severity of the attack. A hot bran mash is suggested for the first meal or two. Then the regular ration should be increased gradually.

Flatulent Colic

Flatulent or wind colic is a distension of the stomach by gas in which the stomach has its capacity increased to a varying extent. This common disorder is generally caused by fermentation of food in the stomach. Moldy or previously frozen foods are most likely to cause the condition. Large amounts of fresh greens or new hay will also contribute to the disorder. Greedy eaters who bolt their food and those with the habit of cribbing are also likely candidates for wind colic.

Symptoms of flatulent colic are generally slow in developing and are rarely so severe as those experienced with spasmodic colic. (On the other hand, flatulent colic is more often fatal.) At first the horse may appear dull. Then he may begin to paw slightly, showing signs of discomfort. The belly gradually enlarges and the flanks become tense and hard. The horse may stand with his back slightly arched and resent being made to move. Breathing becomes labored and the pulse rapid.

At the first indications of flatulent colic, apply hot towels or blankets to the belly, bringing them up over the flanks. Then walk the horse quietly for five minutes and reapply the hot towels. Continue walking the horse and applying hot towels faithfully for thirty minutes. Then, if no gas has been expelled and the flanks have failed to relax, summon a veterinarian at once.

Since horses with flatulent colic are generally quite bloated, it is important that they not be allowed to run or roll. Such actions could prove fatal

Spasmodic Colic

Spasmodic or cramp colic is caused by a spasmodic contraction of the muscular covering of the bowel at some certain point. Unequal distribution of or interference with the nervous supply produces the cramps and therefore the condition is more frequently seen in high-bred or nervous horses. Attacks generally come on quite suddenly.

Spasmodic colic is believed to be caused by indigestible food, drinking large amounts of cold water, and standing in cold rain or drafts of cold air.

Horses suffering from spasmodic colic experience intense though sometimes intermittent pain. During the painless intervals some horses resume eating and appear well until the spasms return. Then all food and even water may be refused. Respirations may become hurried and frequent attempts are made at defecation, which usually results in only small amounts being passed. Similar attempts are made to urinate. The horse lies down frequently, rolls, and looks at his flanks. Acute spasms may bring on a cold, patchy sweat and a rise in temperature.

When spasmodic colic is evident the horse should be warmly clothed and a veterinarian summoned. Horses that become violent from pain should be walked if possible to prevent any injury. If the horse lies quietly it is often best to leave him alone, providing he is not exposed to rain or cold drafts. When the animal will accept food, feed a warm bran mash, warming the water slightly, especially if the weather is cold.

Impaction of the Large Intestines

Impaction of the large intestines is fairly common and, if not promptly recognized and treated, it can result in death. Horses have been known to suffer from impaction for over a week and recover with care and treatment. Few cases last more than four or five days.

Impaction is usually caused by an accumulation of partly digested food or foreign materials (such as sand) which is taken in with food and water over a period of time. Excess bulky food, a lack of water, and insufficient exercise are also contributing factors.

Symptoms of impaction are generally slight abdominal pain in the early stages. The appetite is often lost. Feces are passed frequently, but they are few, small, and dry. As the disorder progresses the horse yawns frequently, paws, and looks at his sides. He may lie down often, flat on his side, with head and legs extended. The intestinal sounds diminish, indicating the absence of bowel movement.

Impactions require the services of a veterinarian. First aid treatment involves walking the horse faithfully for ten minutes every hour. This frequent, mild exercise will help to stimulate the bowel action. Withhold all hay and grain. Feed a warm bran mash with sufficient salt added to encourage the patient to drink more water. Larger amounts of water will generally help soften the impacted mass and hasten its expulsion.

Gastroenteritis

Gastroenteritis, also known as indigestion, is an inflammation of the stomach and intestines which can be acute or chronic. Some horses are naturally endowed with weaker digestive organs and are thus more subject to the condition. The causes of gastroenteritis are generally sudden changes in the diet, irregular feeding, spoiled feeds, and overloading the stomach. Worm parasites—especially strongyles—and sharp teeth are also believed to be contributing factors.

Symptoms of gastroenteritis include irregular appetite; refusing all food at times and eating ravenously at others. Mental dullness, gradual weakness, and a rapid, hard pulse become evident. Movement of the intestines becomes sluggish, and small, shiny-coated manure is passed. Then diarrhea may occur. A considerable amount of sour smelling gas is passed, and colic pain may be present.

The services of a veterinarian are required for treating this disorder as it has many degrees of seriousness, ranking from slight to fatal attacks. The cause of an attack of gastroenteritis should be determined if possible and then corrected to avoid repeated attacks.

Peritonitis

Peritonitis is an inflammation of the membrane lining the abdominal cavity. It is generally caused by injuries, such as puncture wounds of the abdomen, severe blows, or rupture of the stomach. It may also follow a hernia operation or even result from heavy strongyle infestation.

The usual symptoms of peritonitis are gradual dullness, weakness, a high pulse, fever, and shallow breathing. The horse generally stands as the pain is greater while he is down. He walks uneasily, the hind legs moving stiffly. Any pressure on the abdomen causes acute pain, and the animal may bite or kick if touched there. The abdomen is tucked up and accumulating fluid may cause it to be distended considerably.

Peritonitis in horses is generally fatal. If the condition is suspected, contact a veterinarian at once.

Diarrhea

Diarrhea, often due to irritation of the bowels, is quite common in horses. The condition often indicates the body's effort to dislodge indigestible matter, but persistent diarrhea may exist as a complication of a disease.

Diarrhea is often brought on if the horse eats spoiled feed or large amounts of alfalfa, clover, or fresh green grass. Sudden changes in the diet and worms are also believed to be contributing factors.

Symptoms of diarrhea are frequent droppings of a semifluid nature, of a normal or abnormal color and odor. If the condition persists the horse gradually loses flesh and the appetite becomes poor.

In most cases of diarrhea, correcting the diet is all that is required. Eliminate the food causing the condition and give the horse complete rest for 48 hours. Feed lightly and limit the amount of water. Then, if the droppings have not returned to a normal consistency, it is advisable to consult a veterinarian.

Defecation

Normal defecation in the horse occurs eight to ten times in a 24-hour period, the weight varying from 36 to 40 pounds, depending upon the horse's size and the amount of food he consumes. Droppings are often a good indication of the condition of the horse's teeth and digestive system; therefore, the manure should be examined frequently. Droppings filled with unmasticated grain generally indicate that the teeth are sharp or that the horse eats too rapidly. Hard, dry, small droppings often indicate a lack of water or exercise, or indigestible food. This has also been known to be an early indication of pending impaction. Droppings covered with mucus or slime or having an offensive odor indicate the use of too highly concentrated feed or an irritation of the intestines.

Internal Parasites

Parasites of many kinds often reside in the horse. They feed either on tissues of the host or on food which should be available for the nourishment of the horse. Large numbers of parasites can seriously affect the health of the horse and even cause his death. Most parasites (an exception is the BOT) are conveyed to the horse in the food he eats and the water he drinks. Feces of the horse are another source of infestation. Therefore horses confined and fed in a stall or small fenced area are likely candidates for parasitic infestation, because these animals will often become bored and develop the unpleasant habit of eating manure.

There are hundreds of different internal parasites that invade the horse, but only the most common will be described herein.

BOTS

The bot-fly, which somewhat resembles a honey bee, lays its eggs on the various parts of the horse, but particularly on the inside of the knees and about the fetlocks. Although the insect does not sting the horse, the deposition of eggs may create a tickling sensation and cause the horse to toss his head or strike out with the front feet. Some horses have been known to run in an effort to escape the bot-fly.

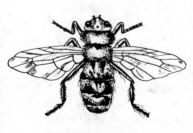

THE BOT-FLY

Once the tiny yellow eggs are laid the bot-fly dies. The eggs remain on the hairs of the horse until they are rubbed by the animal's warm lips or licked by the tongue. This action hatches the eggs and the young larvae enter the horse's mouth, where they remain for two to four weeks. Then the larvae pass into the stomach and intestines, where they attach themselves to the lining for several months. Once

31

fully grown they release their hold and pass out with the feces. The bots then enter a pupal stage for twenty to seventy days before changing into the adult bot-fly. The adult bot-fly is generally seen in late summer or early fall, but this often depends on location and weather conditions. Bot-flys remain active until a freeze.

Bots can cause perforations of the stomach and intestines which may have serious and even fatal consequences. Therefore bot prevention is imperative. All bot eggs on the horse should be promptly destroyed by vigorously applying hot water to them. If the horse is suspected of being bot-infested he should be given a drug that will remove them. This is generally done in the spring and fall. Consult a veterinarian for a bot anthelmintic. A horse infested with bots generally experiences frequent digestive upsets which often develops into colic. There is also lowered vitality and emaciation.

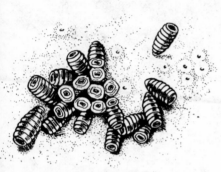

BOTS IN THE STOMACH

STRONGYLES

There are three common species of strongyles which are often found in the horse: *Strongyle vulgaris*, *Strongyle endentatus* and *Strongyle equinus*. These different species vary considerably in size, some being scarcely visible to the naked eye and others reaching a length of two inches.

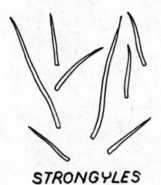

STRONGYLES

The large Strongyle, also referred to as red worms or blood-worms, live in the caecum and colon. Here they produce numerous microscopic eggs, which are expelled with the feces. Within seven to fourteen days the eggs hatch and, when moisture is present, the larvae migrate up the blades of grass and are swallowed by grazing horses.

Horses grazing on permanent pastures are the most likely candidates for strongyle infestation. The infested horse will generally have a poor appetite, a rough coat, tucked-up appearance, anemia, progressive emaciation, and frequent digestive disturbances.

Phenotheazine is agreed to be the most effective drug known at present for removing strongyles from the horse.

ASCARIDS

Ascarids, also known as large roundworms, are the largest and possibly the most common parasites found in the horse. The female roundworm varies in size from six to twenty-two inches long, while the male is from five to thirteen inches long. Fully grown roundworms are generally the diameter of a pencil.

Roundworms are usually found in the small intestines, but they have also been found in the caecum and stomach. In the intestine, the female deposits thousands of tiny eggs which pass out with the feces. Warm, moist weather turns the eggs into embryos, which are swallowed by the horse with food and water. The embryos are liberated in the intestines, penetrating the intestinal walls and entering the blood stream; they then travel to the heart, liver, and lungs. After about a week, the larvae leave the blood stream, travel up the windpipe to the pharynx, and are finally swallowed again to develop to maturity in the small intestine.

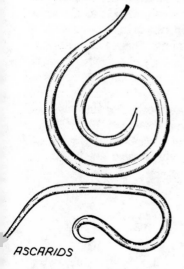

ASCARIDS

Clean paddocks, manure properly disposed of daily, and clean food and water are suggested for the prevention and control of ascarids. Piperazine, thibendazole, trichlorfon, and dichlorvos are drugs that are generally administered for the removal of ascarids from the horse.

Horses heavily infested with ascarids generally cough, and there may be a rise in temperature. The horse is easily exhausted and becomes unthrifty. Frequent digestive disturbances often resemble colic.

PINWORMS

The common pinworms, often seen in the manure of heavily infested horses, are whitish in color and have long slender tails. The females average around one half inch in length, the males are somewhat smaller.

Pinworms are generally found in the caecum, colon, and rectum, but at maturity they usually concentrate in the large intestine. While in the large intestine the females become full of eggs and, when they pass out with the feces, the eggs are deposited around the anal region or in the feces. Once outside the horse the eggs develop and reach the infestive stage within a few days. The horse becomes infested by swallowing the eggs with food and water. The larvae hatch and grow into adults in the intestines.

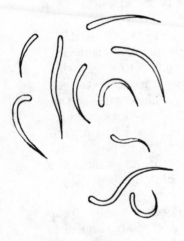

Pinworms can be seen in the feces but another good indication of their presence is the horse frequently backing up against and rubbing on fences or other objects: this indicates the horse's annoyance with the irritation caused by pinworm eggs adhering to the anal region. The irritation often causes restlessness and may result in general loss of condition. Heavy infestation may also cause digestive disturbances and anemia.

Common drugs used for the removal of pinworms are the same as those used against ascarids.

PINWORMS

WORMING

It should be remembered that most drugs used for removing parasites can prove toxic to some horses. Therefore it is a wise practice to give a small dose to begin with. If the new, packaged, do-it-yourself "horse wormers" are used, be sure to read all instructions carefully.

The
Respiratory System

Nose Bleeding, Nasal Gleet, Head Cold, Laryngitis, Roaring, Bronchitis, Lung Congestion, Pneumonia, Pleurisy, Coughing, Broken Wind.

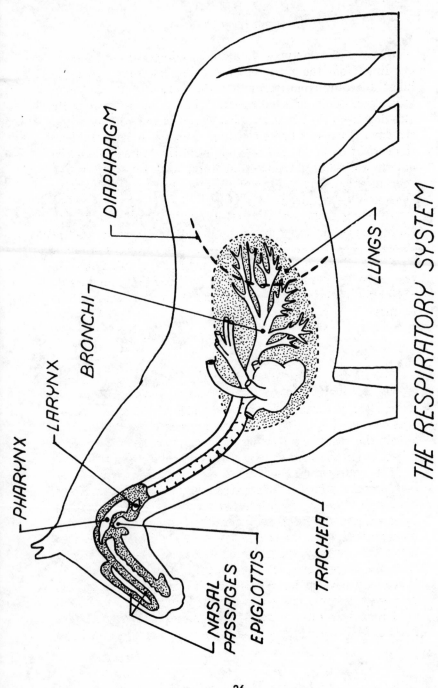

THE RESPIRATORY SYSTEM

PHARYNX

LARYNX

BRONCHI

DIAPHRAGM

LUNGS

NASAL PASSAGES

EPIGLOTTIS

TRACHEA

36

Bleeding from the Nose

There are two types of nasal bleeding seen in horses: bleeding from the nasal chambers and bleeding from the lungs. Bleeding from the lungs is the more serious, as it may indicate a badly affected heart. When a horse is actually bleeding from the lungs, the blood flows from both nostrils in streams. Because a horse bleeding from the lungs can bleed to death if he is allowed to stand still, the animal should be quietly walked until the bleeding diminishes. Contact a veterinarian at once. If the hemorrhage is severe, blood transfusions may be required.

Bleeding from the nasal chambers is rarely serious and the horse may have frequent attacks without great harm. The attacks, though usually unpredictable, often occur after a hard run. Bleeding from the nose may also result from the passage of a stomach tube, especially if the horse resents it. Such bleeding generally is minor and stops within five or ten minutes.

Nasal Gleet

Nasal gleet is the subacute or chronic inflammation affecting one or both nostrils. The condition, which is characterized by a persistent discharge of white or yellowish matter, may be caused by a cold in the head, diseased teeth, an injury within the nostrils, a blow on the head over the sinuses, or a collection of pus in the sinuses or bony cavities in the skull.

The symptom of Nasal Gleet is a discharge from one or both nostrils, which may vary from day to day. Intermittent discharge often signifies infected sinuses. When sinuses are infected, the discharge is generally from one nostril and more profuse when the head is lowered. The bones of the face below the eye may appear to bulge outward and, if tapped with the finger, give off a dull rather than hollow sound. Sores may develop inside the nostrils and often the glands between the lower jaw bones become swollen.

Nasal Gleet often requires the services of a veterinarian. First aid treatment involves keeping the nostrils washed and keeping the discharge cleaned away from manger, feed box, and water containers. Food and water containers should be placed low or on the ground, as discharge is easier when the head hangs down. The horse should be given only very mild exercise until the condition is cleared up.

Cold in the Head

Colds in horses' heads closely resemble colds in humans. They are generally caused by exposure or infection. The condition in itself is not serious, but without proper care it can easily develop into something serious.

Symptoms of a cold in the head are frequent sneezing or snorting. The horse appears dull and there may be a thin discharge from the nostrils, which gradually becomes thick and yellowish in color. The eyes may water and there is often an increase in temperature, a loss of appetite, and a cough.

The horse with a head cold should be warmly blanketed and given complete rest. Fresh air is important, but drafts must be avoided. Particular attention should be paid to the diet. Feed easily digested foods: warm bran mashes, with salt and rolled oats added, are highly recommended. Provide plenty of fresh water. The temperature should be watched carefully as any sudden change, or a fever that does not subside in a few days, may indicate complications.

Laryngitis

Laryngitis is an inflammation of the inner lining of the throat. In humans is is much like a sore throat, but in horses it can assume a more serious phase.

Laryngitis is characterized generally by a slight dry cough which becomes more frequent and harsh, and changes finally to a moist cough. The inflammation of the throat may cause the horse to carry his head stiffly and extended. Any pressure on the larynx induces coughing. Swallowing is often very difficult and in some cases food and water may be returned through the nostrils. The glands between the lower jawbones and below the ears may be swollen. A discharge may appear in the nostrils and, as the condition progresses, breathing becomes noisy and difficult. Fever, loss of appetite, and depression are also common symptoms.

If laryngitis is suspected, it is always wise to contact a veterinarian, as the condition has many degrees of seriousness. First aid treatment involves keeping the horse warmly blanketed and protected from drafts. The throat may be rubbed with liniment. Encourage the horse to take nourishment in the form of bran mashes, linseed gruel, or even fresh grass. Avoid all dry, rough foods. Later, if hay is fed, it should be chopped and moistened with a mixture of molasses and water. All food and water should be offered at a convenient height that will not require the horse to bend his neck. Since lowering the head causes the animal pain, any food placed too low or too high may be refused.

Roaring

Chronic roaring is generally caused by paralysis of the larynx muscles, in most cases the muscles on the left side. It is believed that because the left nerve is much longer and more exposed, it is more commonly affected. Normally the muscles dilate the aperture of the larynx by moving the cartilage and vocal cords outward, which allows sufficient air to pass through. When these muscles are paralyzed the cartilage and vocal cords are allowed to lean into the tube of the larynx; therefore, when the air rushes in, it meets with an obstruction and a noise results.

Roaring is seldom noticed when the horse is at rest, but if the animal is given exercise the characteristic sound is heard. Generally the greater the exertion, the more exhausted the horse will appear. The breathing will become very rapid and difficult, the nostrils will dilate to their fullest extent, and often suffocation will appear imminent.

Once the condition has been definitely established, it generally worsens. There is no preventive treatment. Surgery in the early stages is

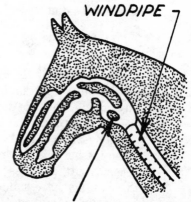

WINDPIPE

THE LARYNX, OR VOICE BOX, IS POSITIONED AT THE END OF THE WINDPIPE.

often successful, but even those horses which are not completely cured are often able to be returned to use.

Bronchitis

Bronchitis is an inflammation of the bronchial tubes and the throat. If the smaller tubes are affected, the condition is serious and could prove fatal, but it is rarely serious when only the large tubes are inflamed. Bronchitis is generally caused by exposure to cold, bacteria, or the inhalation of irritating smoke or chemicals. It also often follows common colds or sore throats.

A horse suffering from bronchitis generally appears dull, the appetite is poor, and breathing is quick and labored. There is usually a harsh, dry cough which increases with any exercise. As the condition progresses, the cough becomes softer and moist, then a nasal discharge appears from both nostrils and the eyes water.

Because it is generally difficult for a nonexpert to discriminate between the two forms of bronchitis (he will also have difficulty in discriminating between bronchitis and pneumonia), a veterinarian should always be consulted. First aid treatment involves covering the horse with a blanket, light or heavy, as the season demands. Give the horse complete rest. Fresh air is essential, but protect against drafts. Provide plenty of fresh water and if the horse retains his appetite a soft, easily digested diet is preferable.

Congestion of the Lungs

Congestion of the lungs is essentially an excess of blood in the lungs. The condition, more common in horses than in any other animal, is due to the inability of the heart to force the blood through the pulmonary vessels.

Congestion of the lungs is generally caused by overexertion when the horse is not in a fit condition. The muscular system becomes soft in horses that stand idle much of the time. When these animals are suddenly given long or hard exercise, they are easily exhausted. The heart and muscles, not accustomed to strain, become unable to perform their work. As a result blood accumulates in the vessels of the lungs and eventually they are engorged with stagnated blood.

This very alarming disorder can prove fatal in some cases. The symptoms generally appear during exercise or shortly afterward. The horse will stand with legs spread out, nostrils dilated, and the eyes staring wildly. The flanks heave heavily and breathing is very rapid. The pulse is weak and rapid. The temperature may rise rapidly and the animal's body may break out in a cold sweat. Death can occur in minutes, but many cases will recover just as fast.

If a horse is being worked hard and suddenly stops, showing signs of exhaustion, discontinue all exercise at once. Cover him with a warm blanket and do not move him for thirty minutes. Then place the animal in a comfortable stall, making sure he is not exposed to any draft. Give complete rest for several days. Feed only easily digested foods. Good care is extremely important, as the condition can be followed by pneumonia. When fully recovered, the horse should receive only moderate exercise for a time, then a gradual increase daily.

Pneumonia

Pneumonia is inflammation of the lungs. It is generally caused by bacteria, exposure to bad weather, and working a horse too soon after illness. A common cold, sore throat, or other illness may be followed by pneumonia if the horse is not properly cared for. The foul air of badly ventilated stables is also known to be a contributing factor.

The earliest symptoms of pneumonia are generally loss of appetite, dullness, and rapid shallow respiration. As the condition progresses the desire for water often increases, and there is a cough and watery discharge from the nostrils. There may be attacks of shivering. The horse with pneumonia will seldom lie down. The condition usually reaches its height in five or six days and then declines in seven or eight days.

When pneumonia is suspected, summon a veterinarian at once. Blanket the horse and place him in a comfortable stall.

Allow plenty of fresh air but avoid drafts. Provide him with plenty of fresh water. The diet should consist principally of bran mashes with rolled oats and salt added. The temperature should be watched carefully. A sudden drop in temperature is a bad sign. Relapses are not uncommon if the horse is returned to work too soon; it is therefore very important to allow sufficient time for a full recovery.

Pleurisy

Pleurisy is an inflammation of the pleurae or membrane coverings of the thorax and lungs. In health this very thin shiny surface is always covered with moisture, which prevents friction between the lungs and the walls of the chest. If it were not for the moistness of the surface of the pleurae, the continual movement and rubbing of parts during inhaling and exhaling would create serious friction. The important moisture is of course absent in pleurisy.

Pleurisy is generally caused by bacterial infection, an injury through the chest wall, or a fractured rib. It may also be a complication of pneumonia. The horse with pleurisy generally loses his appetite and appears distressed, in pain, and not inclined to move. If made to move he may groan. The respiration becomes accelerated and difficult. The temperature will be high and there may be a discharge from the nostrils and eyes. Pleurisy is serious and may prove fatal. Therefore, if the condition is suspected a veterinarian should be consulted at once. Warmly blanket the horse and place him in a comfortable stall free of drafts. Provide plenty of fresh water and feed only easily digested foods.

Coughing

Coughing is a sudden expulsion of air from the lungs. It is a reflex action generally resulting from irritation of membranes of the larynx, bronchial tubes, or lungs. The condition is not a disease in itself, but is generally a symptom of a disorder.

Coughing, which has many forms, may last but a few days or become chronic and persist for months or even years. Indigestion, sore throat, worms in the intestines, bronchitis, heaves, pneumonia, dusty feeds, and poorly ventilated stables are all common causes of coughing in horses.

Proper treatment in cases of coughing depends on the correct diagnosis of the actual condition of which the cough is a symptom.

Broken Wind

Broken wind, commonly known as heaves, is a chronic respiratory condition which involves the overdistention and breakdown of air vesicles of the lungs. When the horse breathes in, the air goes through the bronchial tubes into air sacs which expand, enlarging the lungs and chest cavity. With expiration the muscles of the ribs draw the sacs toward each other, making the chest cavity smaller. This action assists in pressing air out of the air sacks and also helps minute muscles surrounding the air tubes to contract. When heaves develop the walls of the air sacs thicken and lose their elasticity and cannot properly collapse. The minute muscles of the bronchioles become paralyzed and the tubes are unable to contract. The condition therefore allows the air to enter the lungs freely, but breathing out is extremely difficult and added action of the abdominal muscles is required.

Broken wind is generally caused by the regular feeding of dusty foods, or food that is bulky, dry, and unnourishing. Confinement in a poorly ventilated stable and continued hard work that causes severe effort in breathing are also contributing factors.

Symptoms of broken wind are generally doubled expiratory effort and a cough. Watching the flanks will show that the horse appears to heave twice on exhalation. The cough, dry and frequent, often becomes worse with exercise. The condition and general shape of the horse gradually changes. He develops an unthrifty appearance, the stomach enlarges, and the flanks fall away.

There is no known cure for broken wind, but special feeding will ease the condition. This requires elimination of all dust from the feed and a reduction of roughage. All hay should be chopped and sprinkled with a mixture of molasses and water. Hay-grain pellets have been found quite satisfactory for feeding horses with respiratory disorders.

The Nervous System

Blind Staggers, Concussion, Grass Staggers, Cerebral Meningitis, Stringhalt, Shivering, Sunstroke.

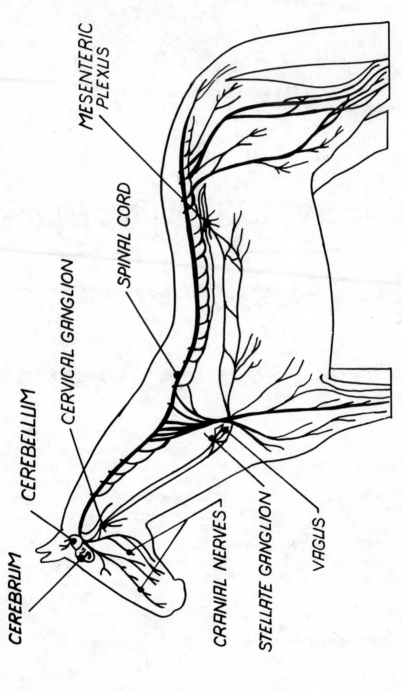

CEREBRUM

CEREBELLUM

CERVICAL GANGLION

SPINAL CORD

MESENTERIC PLEXUS

CRANIAL NERVES

STELLATE GANGLION

VAGUS

THE NERVOUS SYSTEM

Blind Staggers

"Blind staggers" or "congestion of the brain" are names given to an affliction of the brain which causes loss of equilibrium. The disorder is often due to poor circulation caused by a weak heart or undue pressure from a throatlatch or collar.

Symptoms of blind staggers usually appear while the horse is being worked. The animal may stop suddenly, eyes staring. His breathing becomes rapid and noisy. He may sway, stagger, and fall to the ground unconscious. Some horses go into violent convulsions and die, while others regain consciousness within a few minutes. Those who do recover generally show weakness and unsteadiness for several days.

If a horse has a sudden attack such as that just described, remove all tack at once and apply cold water to the head. Have the animal checked by a veterinarian as soon as possible.

Concussion

A concussion is generally caused by a severe blow to the cranium which bruises, or partially destroys the brain.

Symptoms of a concussion are generally present immediately after the injury, but in some cases they may not appear for some time. The horse falls to the ground unconscious and consciousness may not return for some time. The pupils are dilated and breathing is laboured and irregular. Action of the bowels and bladder is generally involuntary. A severe concussion may result in death, while paralysis may occur in some cases after the horse regains consciousness.

A horse suffering from a concussion must be kept as quiet as possible. Ice packs or cold water may be applied to the head and spine as first aid treatment, but a veterinarian should be contacted at once. Horses with even slight concussions should not be worked for two or three weeks.

Grass Staggers

Grass staggers, also termed sleepy staggers and cerebrospinal meningitis, is generally caused by a poisoning and depression of the nervous system from the animal eating food or drinking water containing poison generated by bacteria. Severe grass staggers has three forms:

1. Symptoms of generally fatal attacks are extreme weakness, staggering gait, partial or total inability to swallow, impaired vision and twitching of body muscles. As the disorder progresses the pulse is variable and at times almost imperceptible. Respiration is quick. The temperature does not generally rise, but may drop below normal. These symptoms are usually followed by paralysis of the entire body. With delirium the horse may become violent, but usually a deep coma renders him quiet until death occurs. Death in these cases often occurs within four to twenty-four hours from the time the symptoms become evident.

2. In the second form of grass staggers, from which recovery is often doubtful, there is difficulty in swallowing, a slowness in chewing any food, general weakness, and a slow pulse. But there is generally no evidence of pain. Respiration is usually unchanged, but the temperature may be below normal. These symptoms may remain unchanged for two or three days, after which there is usually either a gradual improvement or a turn for the worse. Cases which take a turn for the worse grow more uncertain in gait, and the pulse becomes slow and weak. Rigidity of the muscles or cramp of the neck and jaws are often evident. Soon there is an inability to stand, and the horse may go into a coma. Death may occur within a few hours or take days.

3. The mild form of grass staggers generally causes only slight weakness and, although swallowing may be difficult, the ability to swallow is never completely lost. There is no fever or evidence of pain and general improvement of the horse is usually evident in about four days.

If grass staggers is ever suspected, contact a veterinarian at once. There is little the inexperienced can do except place the afflicted horse in a comfortable stall and blanket him if the weather is cold.

Cerebral meningitis is a condition in which the vascular membranes enveloping the brain and spinal cord become inflamed.

The earliest symptoms of cerebral meningitis are generally excitement and erratic actions. The horse may blunder over objects, move in circles, and carry his head to one side. Some cases appear dull, staggering in gait, and will move only when made to do so. Respiration in the excited horse is usually accelerated, while in the dull ones it may be irregular in frequency. Spasms of the head, neck, and leg muscles may be evident, and often there is a gradual paralysis of certain muscles. The course of cerebral meningitis is variable, but it should always be considered serious, as it is often fatal.

If cerebral meningitis is suspected, place the horse in a quiet, comfortable stall and contact a veterinarian at once.

Stringhalt

Stringhalt is a disease which causes an involuntary movement of one or both hind legs; although it is classified as a nervous disease, the actual cause is not known.

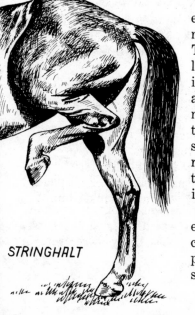

STRINGHALT

The sole symptom of stringhalt is exaggerated hock action, which may not be present at every step. This spasmodic lifting of the hind legs may disappear while the horse is being worked, only to reappear after a short rest. It is often most noticeable when the horse is made to back up or when he is turned sharply. In some cases the spasms may be so acute or convulsive that the animal's usefulness is greatly impaired.

Treatment of stringhalt is generally unsatisfactory, but a surgical operation performed by a competent veterinarian is sometimes successful.

Shivering

Shivering is a nervous disease characterized by involuntary and spasmodic muscular contractions which generally attack the hind legs. The true cause of this disorder is not known, but in some cases it has followed an attack of influenza or strangles.

The progress of Shivering is generally quite slow; long periods may elapse between symptoms. A characteristic symptom of this disease is the frequent lifting of a hind leg. The limb is semi-flexed and abducted, shivering in suspension. The superficial muscles of the thigh and quarter may quiver. If the horse is excited or made to move over quickly, symptoms will often occur. Backing is often difficult.

There is no known cure for shivering and generally the condition worsens, with an increase in frequency and severity of the spasms.

Sunstroke

Sunstroke is a severe nervous disturbance caused by exposure to direct rays of the sun during extremely hot weather.

In sunstroke the nerve centers first become exhausted from overstimulation caused by exposure to heat. Then they become insensible to stimulus and there is a sudden rise in temperature. The temperature may rise to such a degree that the actions of the heart and lungs are either greatly reduced or greatly increased.

A horse suffering from sunstroke will generally appear greatly distressed, stagger, and finally fall to the ground. Some cases lose consciousness, while others may struggle convulsively, making frantic efforts to rise. These cases generally suffer paralysis of the hind quarters. The temperature is high, breathing is shallow and quickened. The eyes stare and the body may be covered with perspiration. In severe cases the body muscles will often be in a state of continued tremor. Death may occur within a few hours where convulsions and paralysis are present. Those cases which lose consciousness and remain quiet are generally the most likely to recover.

When a horse suffers a sunstroke quickly begin bathing the entire body with cold water, particularly the head, neck, and spine. Ice packs applied to the head and neck are greatly beneficial. Protect the horse from the sun. Improvise an awning above him if necessary. Continue the cold water and ice treatment until the temperature drops. Then rub the legs and body vigorously. Once the horse is able to be moved, he should be placed in a comfortable stall and given complete rest. Provide fresh water and feed lightly. Bran mashes are suggested for the first few meals.

Once a horse has suffered a sunstroke, it must be remembered that he is prone to a second attack; he must therefore be provided with ample shade during hot weather.

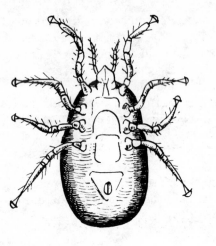
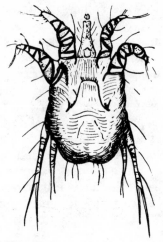
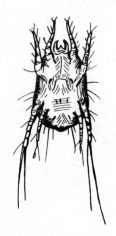
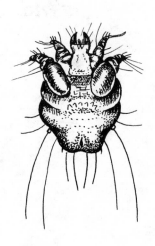

MITES THAT INFEST THE HORSE

The Skin

Mange, Ringworm, Lice,
Nettlerash, Warbles, Hide
Bound, Dandruff, Mane
And Tail Eczema.

Mange

Mange, a contagious disease produced by tiny parasitic arachnids called mites, has two chief forms. Sarcoptic mange is caused by burrowing mites, while psoroptic mange is caused by mites that bite and suck blood. The sarcoptic form is the more serious because the burrowing mites secrete an irritating poison.

Mange generally appears first upon the neck, shoulders, or head, but it may affect any part of the horse's body. The condition may spread over the body until the horse is practically denuded of hair. There is considerable itching and the skin gradually becomes inflamed and swollen. Fluids may ooze from the skin at various locations. As the disease progresses the skin becomes scurfy and it may lay in thick folds. Constant rubbing and biting may produce many open sores which often become infected. Severe cases of mange are generally difficult to clear up and in old or weak horses it may prove fatal.

If mange is suspected, isolate the horse at once and contact a veterinarian, as the disease generally requires skilled attention. Any horse who has had mange should be kept under close observation for some time, as a recurrence of the condition is common.

Ringworm

Ringworm is a contagious disease of the skin caused by microscopic fungi. The condition may be spread directly from horse to horse or through contaminated fences, stalls, grooming utensils, or riding tack.

Characteristic symptoms of ringworm are the round, scaly areas almost devoid of hair. These spots generally appear on the head, on the sides of the neck, and at the base of the tail. Gradually they may spread to any part of the body. A crust may form on the spots and the skin will have a gray, powdery appearance. The oldest part of each spot is its center: the disease spreads from the edges. Often the center heals while the edges are still active and rapidly forming spores.

54

There is generally mild itching accompanying the disease.

If ringworm is suspected, isolate the horse at once. Proper treatment will generally require the skilled attention of a veterinarian. Complete recovery from ringworm takes considerable time.

Lice

Lice are tiny, flattened, wingless insect parasites which are most commonly found during the winter months on ill-nourished and neglected horses. Lice may be spread by direct contact between horses or by infested equipment or stables.

Although lice are extremely small and often impossible to see with the naked eye, their effects are easily recognized. Lice cause their host intense irritation, extreme restlessness, and a loss of condition. The infested horse will frequently scratch, rub, and bite at his body, gradually forming scabs and bald spots. The hair becomes rough and dull. Close examination of the horse's body under warm sunlight will often reveal the tiny lice moving about at the base of the hair.

Infested horses should be isolated and treated. Rotenone or pyrethrins sprays are generally used to destroy lice, but it is wise to consult a veterinarian before administering any treatment.

Nettle Rash

Nettle rash is not a disease but an allergic skin disorder in which round elevations or swellings appear on the body at various locations.

Symptoms of nettle rash are the sudden appearance of swellings that may vary in size from that of a pea to several inches. These raised areas, which may appear on any part of the body, are flat on the surface but elastic to the touch. When the eyelids are affected, they are swollen and puffy in appearance. There is rarely any irritation caused by the condition and in most cases the swellings disappear as suddenly as they appeared.

Nettle rash seems to be most common in idle horses who

are receiving a working ration. Therefore a reduction in grain and any heating foods is suggested. Bran mashes will encourage the elimination of the allergen.

Warbles

Warbles are not infectious, nor a disease; they are actually maggots of the warble fly. The round, firm lumps are commonly found on the muzzle, but may appear on any part of the body.

The lumps, which generally grow larger in the spring or early summer, are caused by a maggot which developed from tiny eggs laid by the warble fly during the previous summer. Warbles will seldom cause a problem unless located under the saddle. In such cases maturity may be hastened considerably by warmth. Hot fomentations of antiphlogistine will bring the warble to a head quickly. When the maggot is ripe a small hole will appear in the center of the lump. The maggot can be pushed through this opening by carefully squeezing on each side of the lump with the thumbs. Any undue pressure should be avoided, as the maggot may burst under the skin, and then the dead tissue may have to be removed by a veterinarian. Once the maggot has been removed, wash the cavity with a diluted disinfectant and then paint with iodine.

Hidebound

Hidebound is not a disease, but is generally an indication or symptom of a disorder or undernourishment. The fatty tissues lying between the muscles and the under surface of the skin are absorbed and lost. The horse affected is generally thin and the hide is tightly stretched over the bones, not easily picked up between the thumb and fingers as with a healthy horse. The hair, usually dull and rough, may fall out, leaving bald spots of various sizes. Dandruff may be thick through the hair and any wounds are generally very slow in healing.

Hidebound may be caused by an inflammation of the stomach and intestines, a chronic case of heaves, worms, underfeeding or old age. To treat Hidebound, the cause must first be found and treated. Then the horse should be fed a diet high in protein. When available fresh green grass should also be fed.

Dandruff

Dandruff, a condition in which the skin becomes scaly, is often caused by a lack of grooming or exercise. Digestive troubles, worms, and a poor diet are also believed to be contributing factors. Baths with medicated soap, frequent grooming, sufficient exercise, and a proper diet will generally help to eliminate most cases of dandruff. A generous amount of linseed meal mixed in the grain ration for a time, and a pound of carrots daily, will be very beneficial.

Mane and Tail Eczema

Mane and tail eczema is essentially a dermatitis that is generally attributed to dirt and neglect. Wet weather often causes maceration of the skin and thus facilitates the entrance of infection.

Symptoms of this skin disorder often escape detection until the condition is already in the advanced stages. The skin of the affected areas becomes thick, scaly, and itchy, and small ulcers may be present. Exudation generally occurs, causing the hair to stick together. As the condition progresses the skin becomes wrinkled and hard. This form of eczema often becomes chronic and is rather difficult to cure.

The first step in treating mane and tail eczema is to clip the hair from the affected areas and then wash the areas with a mercurial type soap. Dry the areas well and then apply an astringent ointment. All heating foods should be greatly reduced and bran mashes fed frequently.

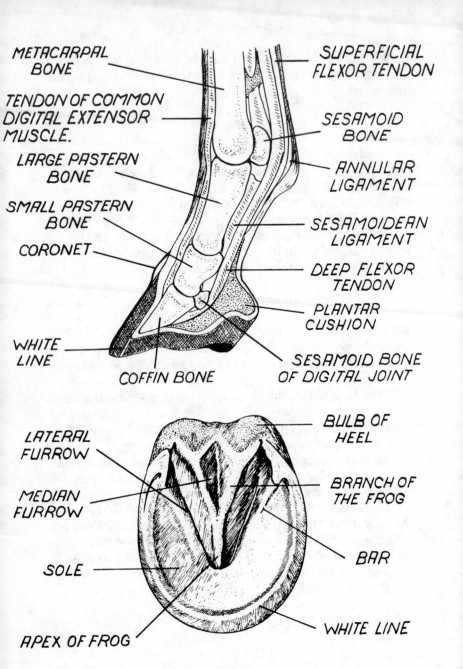

METACARPAL BONE

SUPERFICIAL FLEXOR TENDON

TENDON OF COMMON DIGITAL EXTENSOR MUSCLE.

SESAMOID BONE

LARGE PASTERN BONE

ANNULAR LIGAMENT

SMALL PASTERN BONE

SESAMOIDEAN LIGAMENT

CORONET

DEEP FLEXOR TENDON

PLANTAR CUSHION

WHITE LINE

SESAMOID BONE OF DIGITAL JOINT

COFFIN BONE

BULB OF HEEL

LATERAL FURROW

BRANCH OF THE FROG

MEDIAN FURROW

BAR

SOLE

WHITE LINE

APEX OF FROG

THE HOOF

58

The Feet And Legs

Dry Feet, Navicular Disease, Founder, Quittor, Thrush, Canker, Corns, Quarter Cracks, Contracted Heels, Scratches, Sidebones, Ringbone, Splint, Bowed Tendon, Windgalls, Capped Elbow, Curb, Bone Spavin, Bog Spavin, Thoroughpin, Capped Hock, Lymphangitis, Stifle Lameness, Dislocated Stifle, Rheumatism, Fractures.

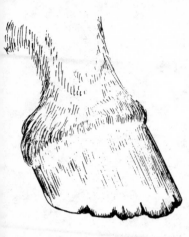

When the horses hooves become brittle from lack of moisture, they not only become more susceptible to disease, but their normal growth is also retarded.

Hoof dryness, most common during the summer months, can almost always be avoided if a good hoof dressing is used frequently. Those dressings containing petrolatum or grease should be avoided. Because greasy hooves cannot absorb moisture, such applications often make dry hooves worse. Cod liver oil and unboiled linseed oil have been used for generations as satisfactory hoof dressings.

Dry hooves may normally be corrected by soaking them in water for five or six hours a day. Another effective method is to attach felt soaking boots to the hooves and keep them wet. Once the hoof has absorbed sufficient moisture, discontinue the water treatment and apply cod liver oil or linseed oil to the hooves with a brush. Be sure to apply the oil to the coronary band as well as the walls and soles. This important area is often overlooked.

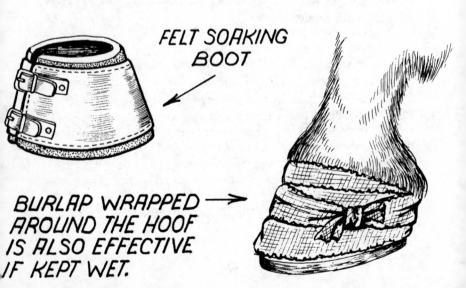

FELT SOAKING BOOT

BURLAP WRAPPED AROUND THE HOOF IS ALSO EFFECTIVE IF KEPT WET.

Navicular Disease

Navicular disease is one of the most serious disorders to which a horse's foot can be subjected. The disease is usually the result of long continued use on hard surfaces or fast paces. It occurs most frequently in the front feet.

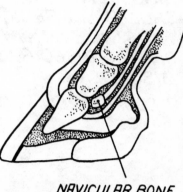

NAVICULAR BONE

Navicular disease is an inflammation of the small navicular bone and the part of the tendon that comes in contact with it. Sharp, bony tumors develop on the bone, causing the horse considerable pain. As the disease progresses, parts of the navicular bone and its surroundings die or become necrotic.

In the early stages of this disorder, symptoms are often obscure. The first indication of apparent trouble is the horse's uneasyness on his front feet. A careful examination may reveal heat in the heels and frog. As the disease progresses, the frog shrinks in size and the heels contract. Progress of this disorder is normally slow, but sooner or later the surgical operation of un-nerving will be required. Satisfactory results from such operations are, however, uncertain.

Soft ground or bedding and cold water bandages tied loosely around the coronet will help reduce pain in a foot affected with navicular disease.

Founder

Founder or laminitis, another serious disorder of the foot, is actually a disturbance of the blood circulation to the feet. Because the horse's hoof and sole are unable to expand to any degree, any abnormal increase in blood circulation means pressure and considerable pain. The degree of such a disturbance of circulation will vary with the cause, and the effects, therefore, may be extreme or so mild that they may not even be noticed.

Founder, which affects the front feet more than the back,

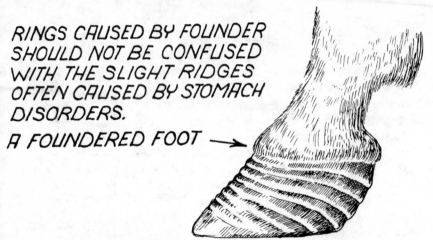

RINGS CAUSED BY FOUNDER SHOULD NOT BE CONFUSED WITH THE SLIGHT RIDGES OFTEN CAUSED BY STOMACH DISORDERS.

A FOUNDERED FOOT →

has various causes. Some believe that too much heating food, prolonged standing on hard surfaces, or drinking considerable amounts of cold water when overheated will contribute to founder.

Founder often comes on quite suddenly. The affected horse will resent being moved and, as his temperature rises, breathing may become hurried. The appetite usually diminishes and the thirst increases. The affected foot (or feet) is hot to the touch and the horse may go down to get the weight off his feet. These symptoms may last as long as four or five days and the condition will become chronic if prompt treatment is not given.

As the disorder progresses, pain and lameness will gradually disappear, but the foot gradually changes in structure. Successive rings appear on the walls and the entire hoof becomes deformed by a bulging sole.

To help relieve the pain of founder, place the affected foot in hot water (up to the fetlock) for at least one hour and then in cold water. Place ice in the water to keep it cold. This treatment should be continued until the pain subsides. Provide plenty of clean bedding and encourage the horse to lie down. Feed bran mashes. The services of a veterinarian are often required in severe cases to give the horse injections of adrenaline.

Quittor is a fistulous sore that is normally located on or just above the coronet. The condition is caused by anything that creates an inflammation inside the horse's hoof. This dis-

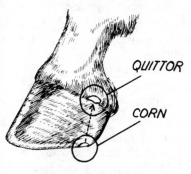

QUITTOR

CORN

order may result from a puncture wound in the sole of the foot, a suppurating corn, or a "close nail."

Quittor is normally recognized by a running sore which appears to heal for a few days and then begins discharging again. In its early stages, a swelling usually appears above the coronet and may spread up the leg. A slight lameness may be noticed before the disorder is

definitely identified, and as the condition progresses, the horse may refuse to place weight on the affected foot.

Surgical attention is usually required to allow free drainage and remove dead tissue. When the location of quittor has been determined, gently pare through the sole of the foot with the curved tip of a hoof knife. When the vent is reached, pus will discharge, relieving pain. The open cavity should be cleaned with an antiseptic and then packed lightly with cotton and bandaged to keep out any dirt. Change the dressing frequently. Also be sure to keep the fistulous sore on the coronet clean by washing frequently with antiseptics.

Thrush

Thrush is a disease of the soft part of the hoof, principally the frog. The disorder is usually caused by the horse standing for long periods in manure and urine-soaked bedding.

Thrush is usually recognized by a discharge of dark, foul-smelling matter from the clefts of the frog. The horn becomes soft and old layers may be lifted off, sometimes exposing the fleshy frog covered only by a thin layer of soft horn. Once the condition is in the advanced stage, the entire hoof is hot to touch, and lameness is more pronounced. This disorder can attack one or more feet at the same time.

In treating thrush, gently pare away the rotten horn and then wash the foot thoroughly with warm soap and water. Apply antiseptics and then pack the clefts of the frog with oakum. Repeat this treatment daily until all discharge has stopped.

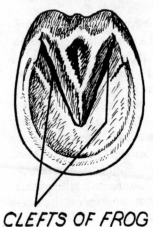

CLEFTS OF FROG

Canker

Canker is a condition similar to thrush, and, like thrush, it is usually caused by unsanitary conditions. Dampness and mud also create favorable environments for the disorder. Canker is generally found in one foot at a time, but it has been known to attack two or all four feet at the same time.

Canker differs from thrush because it not only destroys the sole and frog, but also prevents growth of healthy horn by setting up inflammation in the deep tissue. This disorder actually excites tissues to produce imperfect horn rather than destroying the tissue's power to produce new horn.

Characteristics of canker are usually an extremely offensive odor, a watery discharge from the clefts of the frog which later forms into a yellowish mass, and the rotting away of horn, sole, and frog. The living tissue becomes swollen, dark, and covered with thready horn. Lameness is gradual, but as the condition progresses, it becomes very severe.

The foot affected with canker should be washed thoroughly with warm soap and water. The diseased horn should be carefully pared away and the edges of the healthy horn pared thin to prevent swollen tissue from overlapping. Pack the foot with oakum saturated with an antiseptic, then bandage. When the dressings are changed, any pieces of new horn should be carefully rubbed off with a clean cloth. Once the soft tissues become horned over, discontinue the antiseptics and use a dry germicidal.

Corns

Corns are normally caused by an injury to the sensitive sole of the foot. They are usually, though not always, found in the front feet.

There are three types of corns: dry corns, moist corns and suppurative corns. The dry corns are easily recognized by the appearance of blood-stained horn and the usual absence of inflammation, while the moist corns are characterized by a large amount of inflammation caused by accumulated fluid around the corn. With suppurative corns, lameness is usually intense, but normally subsides once the abscess is opened. A horse suffering with corns will usually advance the affected foot so that it is relieved of all weight. Lameness is most noticeable when the horse is ridden on hard or rough surfaces.

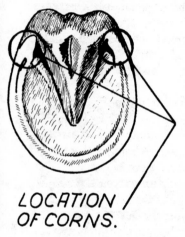

LOCATION OF CORNS.

Treatment of both dry and moist corns involves removing the shoe and cutting away the blood-stained horn. If pain is indicated, soak the foot in cold water at frequent intervals for three or four days. A felt soaking boot would be beneficial, provided it is kept wet. Antiseptic poultices may also be used and are suggested for suppurative corns. Suppurating corns are treated as just described, but surgery may be required to establish drainage. The surgical opening should be carefully covered to prevent any dirt from entering.

Quarter and Toe Cracks

The most common causes of cracks are a lack of frog pressure, excessive trimming of the heels, and excessive dryness of the hoof. Cracks are rarely seen in hooves that are kept moist or in horses that are ridden over soft ground. The seriousness of a crack depends upon its depth. Quarter cracks do not normally extend through the horn to the sensitive tissue, but a toe crack may reach the sensitive lamina and cause severe lameness. The difference between a quarter crack and a toe crack is their movement: toe cracks remain closed when weight is placed on the foot and open when the foot is raised, while quarter cracks work in the opposite way.

These unsightly and often painful cracks in the hoof normally will cause some lameness, which becomes intensified if the horse is made to trot or travel over hard ground. If the crack is deep the opening and closing action, caused by the horse walking, will often pinch the sensitive tissue between the closing edges, thus rupturing small blood vessels. In such cases a constant inflammation results and lameness becomes very severe.

Special shoeing and careful paring of the hoof are usually required to treat both quarter and toe cracks. The entire length of the crack is usually opened with a sharp knife and a V-shaped cut is made to the sensitive tissue beneath. An analgesic ointment is applied to the crack and then it is carefully covered with an oakum pad. The pad may be held in place by wrapping tape around the hoof. This dressing should be replaced as often as necessary and not be left off until the crack has grown together.

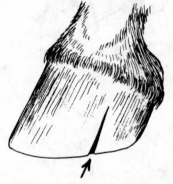

A QUARTER CRACK

Deep cracks in the hoof may require a nail clinch placed midway across the length of the crack to draw it together and prevent further separation.

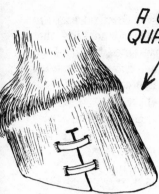

A CLINCHED
QUARTER CRACK.

THE V GROOVE
APPLIED.

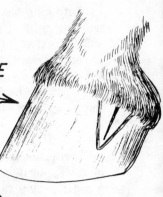

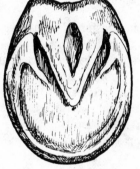

NORMAL
FOOT

Contracted Heels

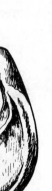

CONTRACTED
FOOT

Contracted heels are usually caused by shoes being left on for long periods and excessive dryness of the hoof. The condition is also encouraged if too much of the frog is cut away so that it does not come in contact with the ground.

A foot with contracted heels will lose its circular shape as the ground surface of the foot gradually becomes smaller than the coronary circumference. The entire hoof also becomes so hard that it is almost impossible to cut with a knife. Lameness is usually quite gradual and often intermittent. It may be noticed most when the horse is ridden on rough or hard ground.

Softening the feet as soon as possible is the first step in treating contracted feet. This may be done by soaking the feet in water for at least an hour a day. Once the hoof is softened, trim the frog lightly and as much from the sole as it will safely stand. Then special shoeing is normally required to spread the heels. The feet should be kept soft by applying cod liver oil or linseed oil to the walls and sole daily.

Scratches

Scratches are generally caused by constant contact with manure and urine or irritating mud. It is also believed that a contributing cause of this disorder may be overfeeding of grain.

The first indication of scratches is a swelling of the bulbs of the heels. Then the skin becomes hot to touch and, as the swelling increases, cracks appear in the skin. The edges of these cracks become inflamed and a thin fluid is discharged. As the condition progresses, the edges of the cracks thicken and ridges of horny scar tissue form. Lameness varies with the degree of inflammation.

To treat scratches, wash the inflamed area with a disinfectant. Then make a pad from clean cotton soaked in a mild disinfectant and place it over the heels. Hold the pad in place with bandages or strips of adhesive tape. Change the dressing twice a day until all swelling subsides.

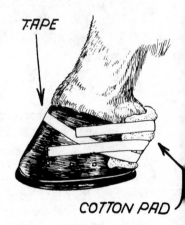

TAPE

COTTON PAD

Sidebones

Sidebones disorder is a serious hardening of one or both of the lateral cartilages. These cartilages, which can be felt by pushing

68

against the skin covering the bulbs of the heels, normally feel elastic, but an inflammation gradually increases their size and finally changes them into hard bones. Sidebones appears most often in flatsoled hooves and in horses that have been worked on hard surfaces. Corns and dry soles are also said to contribute to this disorder. The condition is rarely found in the hind feet.

The horse afflicted with sidebones may or may not be lame. Pressure of the skin against the top of the sidebone may cause pain, and a hard lump and heat may be felt on the coronet on either side of the heel.

Sidebones will usually require the services of a veterinarian. Mild cases may respond to soaking the foot in water to help reduce the fever. Then a special shoe fitted with a rubber pad will be required. Packing the foot with tar and oakum is also helpful to lessen pain and lameness.

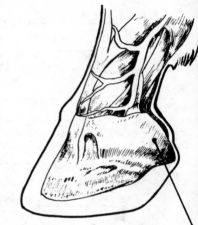

THE LATERAL CARTILAGE

Ringbone

Ringbone is a bone-like growth located anywhere on the pastern bones. The growth may extend almost around the pastern, forming a ring, or it may occur as small bunches on either side or in the front. This disorder may appear in both the front and back legs. This serious disorder is commonly found in horses that have been worked hard in their early life or those whose pasterns are too straight. Heels that are allowed to grow too long may also be a contributing factor.

In the early stages ringbone is

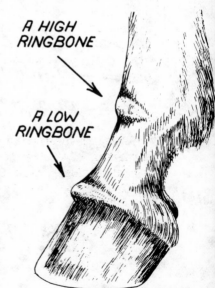

A HIGH RINGBONE

A LOW RINGBONE

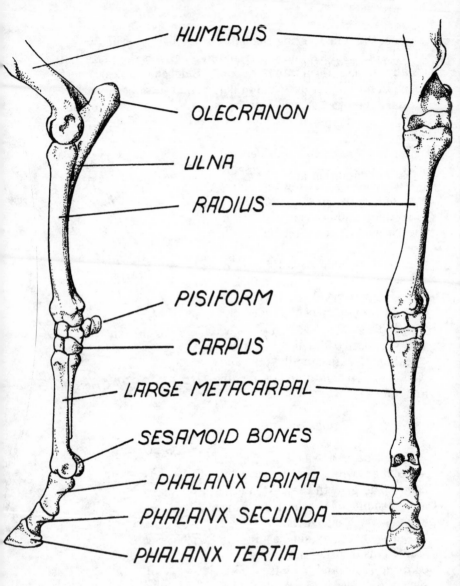

HUMERUS

OLECRANON

ULNA

RADIUS

PISIFORM

CARPUS

LARGE METACARPAL

SESAMOID BONES

PHALANX PRIMA

PHALANX SECUNDA

PHALANX TERTIA

SIDE VIEW

FRONT VIEW

FRONT LEG BONES

usually hard to diagnose, as there is rarely any heat, pain, or swelling; yet lameness is pronounced and constant. It may take weeks before the hard growth can be felt. Sometimes clipping the hair of the pastern will disclose ringbone in its early stages—a soft swelling, sensitive to any pressure.

Treatment of ringbone is always most effective in the early stages, but the prognosis is generally hopeless as far as the horse's usefulness is concerned. The services of a veterinarian are required for ringbone. In some cases, liniment will reduce inflammation and special shoes will help relieve pain.

Splint

A splint is a bony growth which develops on the cannon bone between the knee and the fetlock joint, commonly on the inside of the leg and on the lower third of the principal cannon bone. Splints are of various sizes, ranging from that of a large nut downward to that of a small pea.

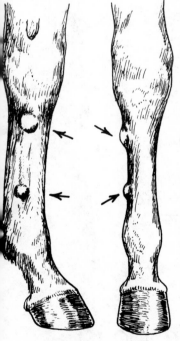

In most instances a splint forms only a single bony growth, but some will pass from the inside to the outside of the cannon bone, between the bone and the suspensory ligament. This type of splint is serious, as it will usually cause permanent lameness. Splints located well forward or low on the cannon bone rarely cause trouble.

This disorder, commonly found in young horses, is normally caused by sprains or injury of the bone and surrounding tissues. Lameness usually accompanies its formation, but subsides once the growth has fully formed. In the early stages there is an increase in temperature over the affected area; pressure will cause the horse pain.

When the splint is first noticed, cold water bandages should be ap-

SPLINTS

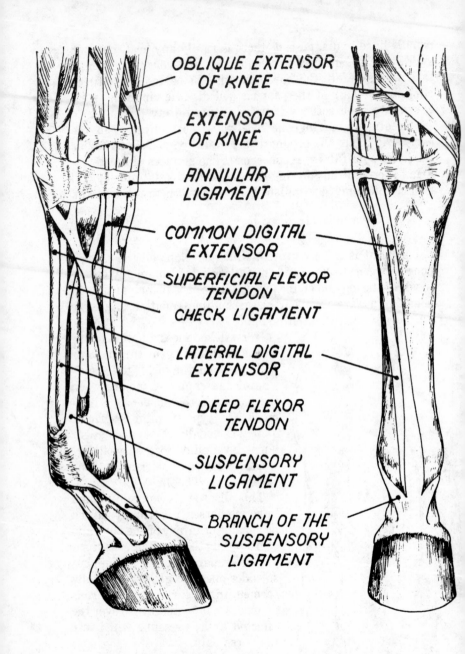

OBLIQUE EXTENSOR
OF KNEE

EXTENSOR
OF KNEE

ANNULAR
LIGAMENT

COMMON DIGITAL
EXTENSOR

SUPERFICIAL FLEXOR
TENDON

CHECK LIGAMENT

LATERAL DIGITAL
EXTENSOR

DEEP FLEXOR
TENDON

SUSPENSORY
LIGAMENT

BRANCH OF THE
SUSPENSORY
LIGAMENT

LIGAMENTS AND TENDONS
OF THE LOWER LEG

plied for at least two days. A good liniment, rubbed well into the skin, will help relieve soreness. Severe splints usually require blistering or pin-firing by an experienced hand.

Bowed Tendon

Tendinitis, more commonly known as bowed tendon, is an inflammation of the large tendons on the back of the leg. The tendons of the front legs are more commonly affected than are those of the back legs. Bowed tendons are usually the result of a severe strain of the fibers making up the tendons, which causes them to be stretched and torn. Horses engaged in racing and jumping are the most susceptible to the disorder.

Lameness is noticed first with bowed tendons, followed by

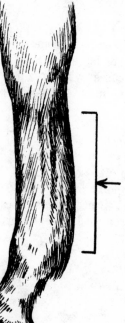

heat, swelling, and sensitivity of the tendon to any pressure. The entire length of the tendon in the cannon area may be affected, or only a small part of it. Symptoms may not be noticed until the day following the accident, or they may appear within a few hours.

Absolute rest is essential for the horse afflicted with a bowed tendon. Cold water or ice water packs should be applied to the leg for the first two or three days, or until the acute swelling and tenderness subside. Then bathe the leg with hot water, dry thoroughly, and massage with a good liniment. After allowing the area to be exposed to the air for thirty minutes, bandage, using a generous supply of cotton under the bandage. Repeat treatment daily. If the condition does not respond to treatment, it is probable that blistering or firing must be resorted to.

Windgalls

Windgalls, or windpuffs, are the result of a severe strain which causes small membranous sacs to become oversized. These sacs normally secrete small amounts of fluid which serves to lubricate joints. Normally only enough fluid necessary to prevent friction is secreted, but inflammation, resulting from concussion, causes the amount to increase and results in a distention which pouches out under the skin in the form of a soft bunch.

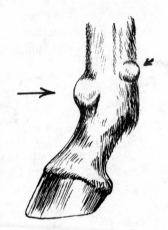

Windgalls, which may appear in both the front and back legs, are usually painless and will not normally cause lameness. If they are struck or bruised, however, acute lameness may result and persist for some time. In most cases, windgalls are best left alone, although blistering or firing may offer good results if done during the early stages.

Capped Elbow

A capped elbow or "shoe boil," as it is often called, is an enlargement which appears on the point of the elbow. It is generally the result of a bruise, and repeated bruising causes a tumor-like growth which may grow to large proportions.

Capped elbows generally result from the heel of the hoof pressing against the elbow when the horse lies down, but another contributing factor is a lack of sufficient bedding in the stall.

In the early stages of this disorder, there will usually be heat and a sensitive swelling. As the swelling increases in size, the free action of the affected leg may be interfered with, but lameness is seldom present.

When first recognized, a capped elbow should be treated with frequent applications of cold water, followed by the use of a liniment

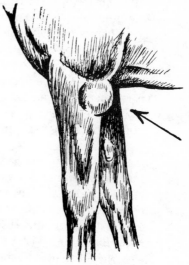

and a brisk massage. A swelling that increases to large proportions will usually contain considerable fluid and it should be lanced by an experienced hand.

Curb

A curb is the result of inflammation causing a thickening or bulging of one or all of the tendons and ligaments on the back of the hock. The normal straight line of the hock (viewed from the side) becomes curved and bulging. Curb can be a serious disorder. It is generally caused by sudden or severe strain, such as that experienced in rearing, jumping, sudden and short stops, hard pulling, and slipping. Some authorities believe that horses with "sickle hocks" or those with weak joints are the most likely to experience curb. Curb is a blemish, but rarely does it cause permanent lameness.

This disorder will normally begin with signs of inflammation within a few hours after the ligament or tendon has been strained. Lameness may be present, but it is often intermittent. A swelling appears, and there may be a varying degree of heat and soreness. The horse may stand with the hock joint bent and if made to move he is inclined to walk on the toe of the affected leg.

The horse suffering with curb should be given complete rest while the affected hock is treated with frequent applications of cold water. Severe cases may require blistering or firing for an effective cure. Obstinate cases may also be helped by using a special high-heeled shoe on the affected leg.

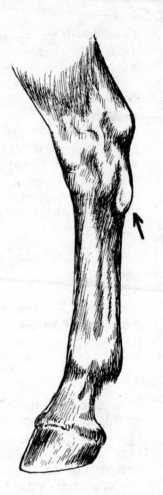

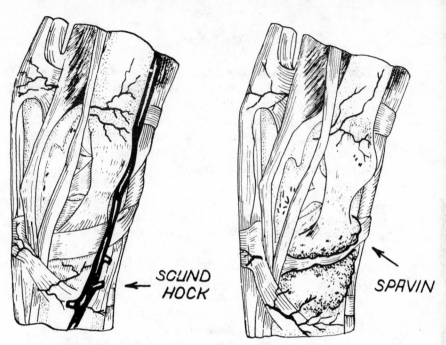

SOUND HOCK

SPAVIN

HOCKS WITH SKIN REMOVED

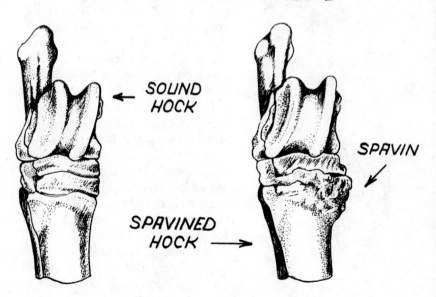

SOUND HOCK

SPAVIN

SPAVINED HOCK →

BONE SPAVIN

77

Bone spavin is a serious disease of the bones of the hock joint which generally causes deformity and permanent lameness. When the synovial fluid that lubricates the joint is broken down by inflammation and carried away in circulation, friction results. This friction stimulates the growth of a bony tumor which causes extreme pain when its sharp edges tear into ligament and tendon coverings.

There are several forms of bone spavin, but the most common involves the cuneiform bones at the front and inner side of the hock. This serious condition is generally caused by a severe strain which tears a ligament or lacerates some of its fibers.

A bone spavin generally develops slowly, so that in its early stages it is often difficult to recognize. Lameness is noticed first. As the condition progresses, the skin over the inside of the hock becomes hot to touch and the area sensitive to any pressure. The bony growth develops until it may be easily seen and felt at the lower front portion of the inside of the hock. The horse will usually stand with the hock bent and the lower part of the leg brought forward, resting on the toe.

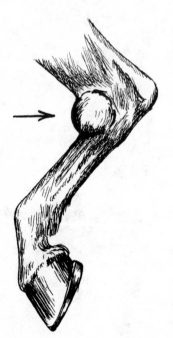

If treated in the early stages, some cases of lameness resulting from bone spavin may respond to treatment, but the bony enlargement usually remains. The horse should be given complete rest for at least two months. Liniments and vigorous massage should be used frequently to increase circulation to the hock joint. Persistent treatment is very important. A special shoe equipped with high heels is also beneficial.

Bog spavin is a soft, puffy swelling located on the inside of the hock. The condition is caused by the inflammation of a joint-oil sac located in the fold of the hock at the front and toward the inner side. Injury causes the oil sac to secrete large amounts of fluid, which stretches the sac walls and results in a large swelling.

Caused by strains or slipping, a bog spavin is generally not easy to recognize until it is well advanced. Lameness and inflammation are observed first and gradually a soft, round bunch develops. This well-defined bunch is usually soft, and the presence of fluid within is easily detected by pressure with the fingers. When the horse places weight on the affected leg, the bunch may appear tight, but when the weight 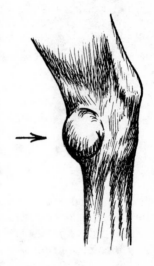 is removed and the hock joint bent, it may appear smaller in size and be soft to the touch.

In treating bog spavin, the horse should be given complete rest for at least three weeks. Liniment applied frequently will help relieve soreness and reduce congestion. Special shoes with high heels may help retard progress of the condition if used in the early stages.

Thoroughpin

Thoroughpin is a soft enlargment located in the hollows at the back of the hock, which may be seen on both sides. The condition is caused by the dilation of the synovial sac, which overfills with lubricating fluid. The enlargement may occur on one or both sides of the hock, but, when found on each side, both parts actually comprise one single enlargement. When

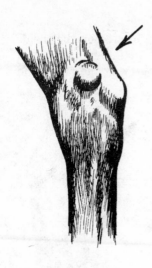

pressure is applied to the swelling on one side, fluid will usually be forced to the other side of the hock, thus making the bunch larger on that side.

This disorder generally appears soon after the injury occurs. A hot, tense, and painful swelling normally develops, but in some cases a dropsical condition may occur instead, with the swelling cold to the touch and not painful. The horse is generally lame and may stand with only the toe touching the ground.

When thoroughpin is first recognized, the horse should be given complete rest and the affected leg should be shod with a special high-heeled shoe. Frequent applications of hot water and liniment are beneficial, but if the swelling does not respond to treatment and subside it gradually becomes chronic.

Capped Hock

A capped hock is actually a bruise, generally caused by repeated kicking against stall walls or a lack of sufficient bedding. The condition may develop into a tumor-like swelling and often assume large proportions.

In the early stages, a capped hock is generally recognized by heat, pain, and a swelling at the point of the hock. As the swelling gradually diminishes, the tissues on the point of the hock may become thickened and toughened. Lameness is seldom present. Liniment and massage will help relieve inflammation and soreness. The cause of the capped hock should be removed and in some cases a protective hock boot should be used.

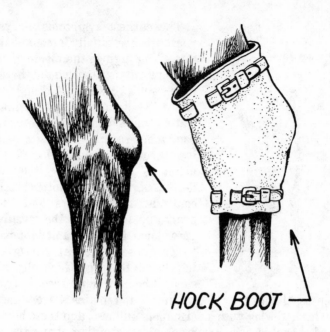

HOCK BOOT

Lymphangitis

Lymphangitis is a specific inflammation of the lymphatic structures which generally affects the hind legs and rarely the front ones.

This disorder, which comes on quite suddenly, is commonly caused by an abundance of food too high in nutrition, long periods of idleness with a heavy food ration, overworking an unconditioned animal, and a lack of care during an attack of distemper or pneumonia.

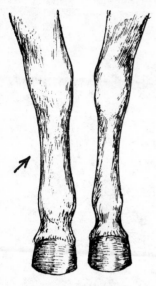

The earliest symptoms of lymphangitis are usually lameness and a swelling high on the inside of the thigh. Within a few hours the leg may swell to twice its normal size and the skin may crack, allowing a watery fluid to discharge. A high body temperature develops, breathing becomes accelerated and the action of the kidneys and bowels decreases. These symptoms may continue for 48 hours and then gradually lessen. As the swelling goes down the pain and lameness lessen, but seldom does all the swelling leave the leg. Generally the slower the horse is to recover from lameness, the larger the swelling that remains. Severe cases often leave the leg with a permanent fullness, and these horses are often subject to recurrent attacks of lymphangitis.

At the first signs of lymphangitis, bathe the entire leg with hot water for 30 minutes, repeating every two hours. Withhold all grain. Feed hot bran mashes and limited amounts of hay. Provide plenty of fresh water. Liniment and massage will help stimulate circulation and relieve swollen lymphatic glands, providing the skin is not broken and discharging serum.

Stifle Lameness

Stifle lameness is the result of a severe strain on ligaments or a bruise near the stifle joint. The stifle joint, formed by the femur, patella and tibia bones, is the largest and most complicated in the horse's structure.

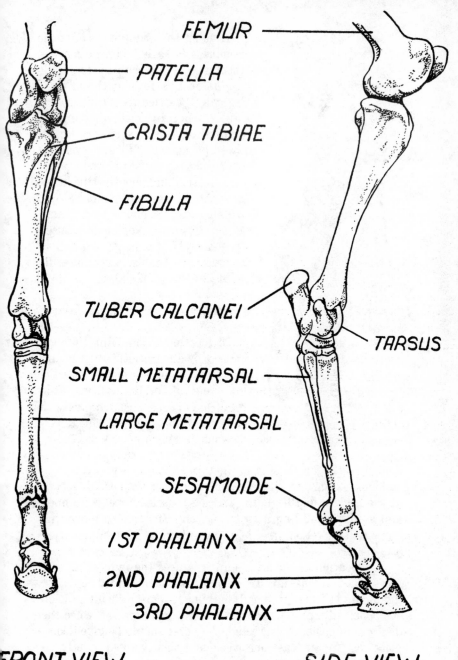

FEMUR

PATELLA

CRISTA TIBIAE

FIBULA

TUBER CALCANEI

TARSUS

SMALL METATARSAL

LARGE METATARSAL

SESAMOIDE

1ST PHALANX

2ND PHALANX

3RD PHALANX

FRONT VIEW

SIDE VIEW

BACK LEG BONES

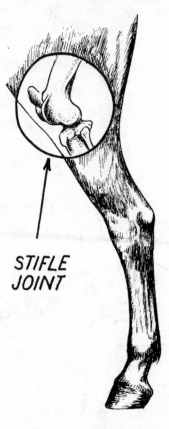

STIFLE JOINT

Among the symptoms of stifle lameness is severe lameness when the horse is made to move. While the horse is standing, the affected leg may be frequently lifted. The hip is generally lowered, the muscles relaxed, and the joints bent. Swelling may be felt and pressure over the area causes pain.

A horse afflicted with stifle lameness should be given complete rest. Applications of hot water gradually changed to cold should be used frequently. Liniment vigorously rubbed upon the skin over the stifle joint is also beneficial.

Dislocation of the Stifle Joint

Dislocation of the stifle joint is caused by the patella slipping upward and becoming locked over the lower end of the femur bone. This condition occurs most commonly in colts or young horses, but it can happen to horses of any age.

Dislocation generally occurs suddenly, as the horse slips or gets up. The affected leg may suddenly become so rigid it cannot be moved forward or bent at the hock and stifle joint. The leg muscles appear cramped and a slight swelling may be present. If made to move, the horse will travel on three legs, dragging the affected leg after him.

Dislocation of the stifle joint requires the immediate services of a veterinarian. If the joint is not promptly replaced, ligaments become stretched, making it more difficult to keep the bone in its proper location after it has been set. Once the dislocation has been corrected, the horse should be given complete rest for at least one week and then walked quietly on level ground. Applications of liniment during this time are beneficial for increasing circulation and helping to restore vitality to injured muscles and ligaments.

Rheumatism

Rheumatism indicates disease of muscles, tendons, joints, and nerves. It generally occurs quite suddenly and although it is most common in older horses, those of any age are susceptible. Dampness and humid atmospheres, exposure to cold, and sudden changes in temperature are believed to be contributing factors to rheumatism.

Symptoms of rheumatism are generally pain in the muscles, ligaments, and tendons. Stiffness and lameness may be present for days or months and then suddenly disappear, only to appear in some other joint or leg. Often a cracking sound may be heard in the joints when the horse moves. The condition may become chronic and joints may be permanently enlarged.

Rest, applications of liniment to affected areas, and a diet of easily digestible food is suggested for the horse afflicted with rheumatism.

Fractures

A fracture is a break in a bone. When a bone completely separates, it is called a complete fracture and when a break extends only partly through a bone it is known as an incomplete fracture. A simple fracture is a break where tissues are not torn and a compound fracture one where they are.

Fractures are serious in the horse because of his large size. In many cases there is no satisfactory treatment and the animal must be humanely destroyed. The location of the broken bone, the horse's age and his disposition generally are factors in deciding the animal's fate. A young horse with a quiet disposition suffering a simple fracture of the lower leg is usually the best prospect for recovery.

Symptoms of a fracture generally vary in accordance with the type of break and its location. Incomplete fractures usually

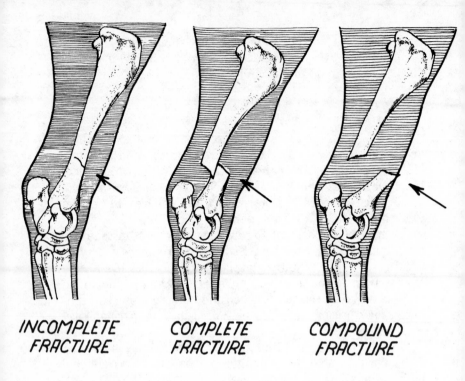

INCOMPLETE
FRACTURE

COMPLETE
FRACTURE

COMPOUND
FRACTURE

cause pain and inflammation, but they are often not recognized unless the crack enlarges and makes a complete fracture. A complete fracture allows abnormal movement of the body or limb. A compound fracture generally shows injury to surrounding muscles, nerves, blood vessels, and skin along with abnormal movement of body and limb.

When a fracture is suspected, the immediate services of a veterinarian are required.

Miscellaneous Diseases

Strangles, Equine Influenza, Swamp Fever, Sleeping Sickness, Glanders And Farcy, Equine Abortion, Tetanus, Malignant Edema, Azoturi, Tick Fever, Hydrophobia.

Strangles

Strangles, also known as distemper, is an infectious disease which is seen more frequently in younger horses. It appears as a fever with the formation of pus in the air tubes and lungs. Frequently abscesses form in various parts of the body. Strangles is generally caused by germs spread through food and water that have been contaminated by the discharges of an infected animal.

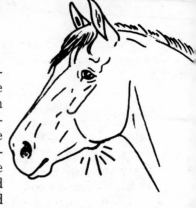

LOCATION OF ABSCESS

Symptoms of this disease generally appear from four to fourteen days after the horse has been exposed to the germs. The horse begins to act dull, his appetite becomes poor, and his temperature will rise considerably. There is a thin, watery discharge from the nostrils which gradually thickens and becomes a yellowish color. Coughing may be frequent and the glands beneath the throat swell and become hot to touch. Movements of the head are painful. Within a few days a large swelling appears near the angles of the branches of the lower jaw. Gradually, one or more soft places are felt beneath the skin covering the swelling. They become moist with a yellowish fluid; finally the skin may burst and thick pus, streaked with blood, is discharged. Once this abscess has ruptured, the horse will show signs of feeling better and the temperature will gradually drop. The average case will recover in two to four weeks, providing there are no complications.

In treating strangles it should be kept in mind that the disease is very contagious and the infected horse should be isolated. Place the warmly blanketed horse in a comfortable stall, well ventilated but free of any drafts. Feed only easily digested foods and provide ample fresh water. The nostrils should be washed frequently with warm water. Antibiotics should be given to fight infection. Frequent bathing of the abscess with hot water will hasten its maturity. Do not open the abscess until it is mature. After recovery the horse should be kept isolated until all discharges cease.

Equine Influenza

Influenza, also known as shipping fever, is an acute, highly contagious disease believed to be caused by germs so small that they cannot be seen with the most powerful microscope. These tiny germs are found in the blood and other fluids within the horse's body.

The disease may be spread through discharges of the eyes and nose and also in the manure. Therefore a healthy horse is infected by eating or drinking after an animal that has the disease.

Early symptoms of equine influenza are generally depression, great weakness, and a loss of appetite. There is a high fever, the heart beats rapidly, and the rate of breathing increases considerably. The lining membranes of the eyelids are swollen and they become a dark pink color. Tears become mixed with pus, which may gather between the eyelids and adhere to the skin below them. There is generally a strong, dry cough which changes to a moist one as the disease progresses. Within a few days diarrhea may develop and symptoms of colic may appear. In some cases the legs and abdomen swell.

Pneumonia and pleurisy are frequent complications in cases of influenza. Therefore a veterinarian should be summoned as soon as the disease is suspected. Isolate the sick horse at once. Keep him warm, but allow plenty of fresh air. Provide ample water and encourage the horse to eat, as the disease is very wasting. Offer easily digested foods, such as bran mashes.

Swamp Fever

Swamp fever is a serious disease of the blood that has three forms varying in course and intensity. The cause of swamp fever is believed to be a specific virus, which may live in its host for years before it is eliminated, probably in some secretion or excretion. Insects are thought to be carriers, as it has been found that the disease is most common where there are biting insects.

Symptoms of the acute form of swamp fever are a sharp rise in temperature, dejection, and the head held low. The legs are weak and the weight is shifted from one leg to the other frequently. The membranes of the eye show considerable congestion and watering. There may be heavy sweating and diarrhea. These symptoms generally last from three to five days and then disappear, but then they are all repeated. The length of time between attacks usually determines the horses chance to survive: the closer together the attacks occur, the less chance the horse has.

Chronic cases of swamp fever are generally weak and sluggish. Considerable weight is lost and anemia is apparent. The heart action becomes irregular and the pulse is slow and weak. The horse moves with a staggering gait. Horses affected with the chronic form may appear to recover, but actually the disease only becomes inactive. Although the animal shows no signs of the disease, the virus is still in his blood. Therefore he becomes a carrier. As a carrier he is a threat to other animals because the infection can be reactivated at any time. Complete recovery is very rare.

Horses who experience the subacute form will have milder

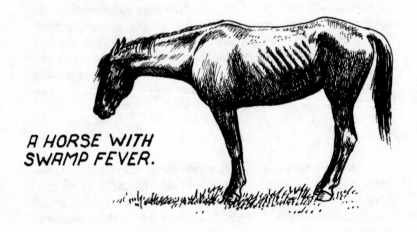

A HORSE WITH
SWAMP FEVER.

90

attacks at longer intervals, but even this form of the disease may become chronic or result in death.

As there is no known cure for swamp fever, it is generally recommended that infected horses be destroyed. If swamp fever is suspected, isolate the animal at once and contact a veterinarian.

Sleeping Sickness

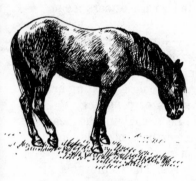

A HORSE WITH
SLEEPING SICKNESS.

Sleeping sickness, also known as equine encephalomyelitis, is an acute infectious disease affecting the central nervous system. The disease may be transmitted to humans. The cause of this highly infectious disease is a filterable virus. which is carried from sick to well animals by mosquitoes.

Early symptoms of sleeping sickness are generally an increase in temperature and drowsiness. The muscles of the head, shoulders, and flanks twitch noticeably. The horse stands with a depressed head and, when he is moved, the gait is staggering. He may walk aimlessly, crashing into objects, and he may grind his teeth frequently. The mouth has a foul odor and food and water may dribble from the mouth and nostrils. The eye membranes appear yellowish or muddy in color. Eating and drinking are difficult. Finally there is an inability to swallow and paralysis of the lips. The horse grows gaunt and eventually he may fall to the ground, unable to rise. At this stage a horse has little hope of recovery and death may occur in a few hours. Those who do survive are likely to have permanent brain damage.

If sleeping sickness is suspected isolate the horse at once and contact a veterinarian. An antiencephalomyelitis serum, if used in the early stages, has saved many infected horses. Horses can be protected from this disease by a vaccine, which should be administered by a veterinarian in the spring or early summer.

Glanders is a highly contagious disease of the lymphatic system which manifests itself in ulceration, nodules, and degenerations in the respiratory passages. Glanders of the skin is called farcy. The cause of both glanders and farcy is contagion by means of the specific virus of the disease. When a horse swallows food or water infected with glanders germs, he becomes infected.

Symptoms of glanders affecting the lungs, which may not appear until weeks or months after exposure to the virus, are coughing and difficulty in breathing. There is generally a noted run-down condition and there may be nose bleeding or a discharge of bloody mucus during spells of coughing.

Nasal glanders usually begins like a cold in the head. There is a watery discharge from one or both nostrils which gradually becomes thick and yellowish in color. Whitish lumps and blood may be mixed in the discharge. The membranes of the nose swell and small grayish lumps appear upon them. These soon break and form ulcers. When these ulcers heal a characteristic star-shaped scar is left.

Symptoms of farcy, or skin glanders, are small swellings which develop in the skin of the legs and under the abdomen. A small round opening generally forms in the skin over the swelling and a sticky, yellowish pus discharges. These openings gradually become larger until the swelling is finally replaced by a sunken ulcer. The horse may have a fever and, as the appetite is lost, the animal becomes thin and weak.

As there is no known cure for glanders or farcy, those animals who survive may be suspected of being carriers of the disease. If the disease is suspected contact a veterinarian at once. A mallein test should be performed to make a positive diagnosis.

Equine Abortion

Equine abortion is the premature expulsion of the impregnated ovum. Abortion can be caused by spoiled feeds, poisonous plants, or injury, but over half the abortions in horses are believed to be caused by bacterial or viral infection. The most common of these are abortion caused by *Salmonella abortivo-equina*, streptococcic abortion and epizootic abortion.

Salmonella abortivoequina is an infectious disease carried by an organism that is believed to enter the mare in the food and water she consumes. Abortion caused by this disease generally occurs from the fourth to eighth month of pregnancy. The mare will often show signs of illness before and after the abortion.

The streptococcic infection, which is believed to occur during service or after foaling, is known to cause abortion at any time during pregnancy, but it is most common in the early months. If abortion does not occur, the foal is generally born infected.

Epizootic abortion which generally occurs between seven and eleven months, is often accompanied by a fever and mild respiratory infection.

Symptoms of abortion will usually vary according to the stage of pregnancy. It is seldom observable during the first two months of pregnancy. Abortion occurring somewhat later in pregnancy will generally cause a loss of appetite, neighing, and considerable straining until the fetus is expelled. Abortion in the later stages of pregnancy will often cause symptoms of normal parturition, except that there is usually more effort and straining required in expelling the fetus. The symptoms may last an hour or they may continue for an entire day.

To prevent the spread of these contagious infections, all vaginal discharges, dead fetuses, and membranes should be quickly buried. The infected mare should be isolated and not bred again until the infection has cleared up. All manure and bedding should be burned or soaked with a strong disinfectant before it is disposed of.

Many cases of abortion caused by infection could be avoided by vaccinating the brood mare each year against salmonella, mating only healthy mares to healthy stallions, and practicing cleanliness at the time of service and examination.

Tetanus

Tetanus, also known as lockjaw, is an acute infectious

disease caused by the bacillus of tetanus. When this bacillus enters the horse's system it produces a deadly poison which acts upon the entire nervous system.

The usual manner in which a horse becomes infected is through a deep puncture wound. Nail punctures in the hoof often result in tetanus mainly because the wound may go unnoticed and does not always receive proper treatment.

In most cases of tetanus, the first symptoms are noticed during the second week after the horse is infected. Muscles of the neck and jaws gradually stiffen. The head is held stretched outward. A characteristic sign of tetanus is the extension of the third eyelid from the corner of the eyes halfway across the eyeball. Eating and drinking become difficult and finally impossible because spasms of the jaw muscles allow only partial opening of the mouth. The horse will generally stand with legs stiff and awkwardly spread. The tail is held high and the ears are rigidly erect. Breathing is fast and difficult. The heart action is quickened. The horse becomes extremely nervous and any noise or sudden movement

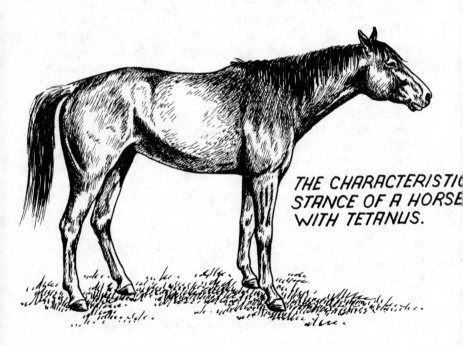

THE CHARACTERISTIC
STANCE OF A HORSE
WITH TETANUS.

may cause convulsive spasms. The stricken animal will generally stand as long as it is possible.

Tetanus can be avoided by immunization with tetanus toxoid. If a horse suffers a deep or puncture wound and has not been immunized against tetanus, contact a veterinarian at once.

Malignant Edema

Malignant edema is an infection caused by a germ called *Clostridium septicum*. The infectious bacteria are believed to live in the soil and enter the horse's system through a wound. The condition may also result from unsanitary conditions during surgery and foaling.

Early symptoms of malignant edema are a hot, painful swelling of the affected area, a high fever, loss of appetite, extreme depression, and labored breathing.

Once the infection is well established there is no known cure. But if it is treated in the early stages, antibiotics have a therapeutic value. Prevention is the best answer. There is a preventive vaccine, and therefore it is wise to vaccinate all horses in areas where the soil is suspected of being contaminated with *Clostridium septicum*. Other preventive measures include treating all wounds, regardless of how minor, sterilizing all instruments used for surgery or for injections, and being sure that parturition takes place in clean surroundings.

Any horse suspected of malignant edema should be isolated. Contact a veterinarian at once. It should also be mentioned here that humans are susceptible to this disease and precautionary measures should be taken.

Azoturia

Azoturia is a disease of which the true cause is not known, but in nearly every case history the horse had been idle and the grain ration not appropriately reduced.

Symptoms of Azoturia generally appear after the horse has been worked for a while. Increased excitability, profuse

AZOTURIA

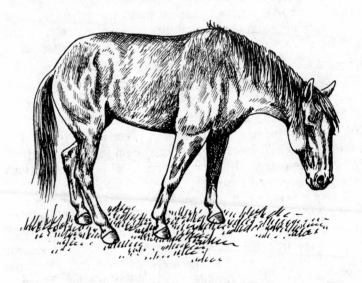

sweating, and rapid breathing suddenly are apparent. Lameness then progresses rapidly and finally the horse begins to stiffen in the hindquarters. He may drag the hind legs and knuckle over in the back fetlocks. The muscles of the croup and loins become swollen and hard. The temperature rises.

When azoturia is suspected, the horse should be placed in a comfortable stall as soon as possible and a veterinarian summoned. Hot blankets may be applied to the loins and then covered with a plastic sheet to keep in the steam. When the blanket cools down, replace with another hot one. This treatment may be required continuously for days, depending upon the severity of the case. All food offered the horse should be of an easily digested and laxative nature.

Mild cases of Azoturia generally recover quickly whereas severe cases can end in death within a few days. Once recovered, the horse should be allowed to develop strength in his legs gradually, without any danger of overexertion. Turning out to pasture for a month generally offers the best results.

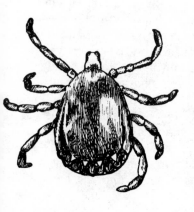

TICK

Horse tick fever is a blood disease brought on by blood parasites. Carried by the tick, these parasites enter the blood stream and destroy the red cells. This disease is most commonly found in hot, humid areas.

Symptoms of Tick Fever are a high temperature, drowsiness, rapid breathing, and accelerated heart action. The hind legs may be swollen and the mucous membranes of the mouth and eyes become pale and turn a yellowish color. Severe cases may collapse after a few days and die.

No treatment has been found to eliminate all the blood parasites once they are established. Horses which have recovered from this disease are believed to be possible carriers.

In areas where ticks are prevalent, there should be a daily inspection of the horse's entire body. Any ticks found should be promptly removed. If tick fever is suspected, or feared, a lab analysis of the horse's blood, or the tick, can lead to a positive diagnosis.

Hydrophobia

Hydrophobia, also known as rabies, is an acute, infectious disease caused by a filterable virus which is carried into a bite wound by infected saliva. This fatal disease is generally transmitted to horses by infected dogs or certain wild animals.

Symptoms of hydrophobia generally appear within 45 to 90 days after the horse is infected, but earlier and later development is common. An early sign of infection is an irritation of the scar which resulted from the infectious bite. The horse may frequently rub or bite at it. The horse is easily frightened and excited. The pupils of the eyes become dilated and there is a staring expression. As the disease progresses the lips contract, exposing the teeth, and foamy saliva drools from the mouth. The horse expresses a great desire to bite and he may attack man or animal. Some cases will bite upon fences or solid walls. Swallowing becomes difficult and any water taken in the mouth may run out the nostrils. Paralysis of the hind legs gradually develops until the horse finally falls to the ground where he usually remains until death occurs.

Any horse suspected of being bitten by a rabid animal should be promptly reported to a veterinarian. The horse who is considered worth the expense should be given the Pasteur treatment shortly after being bitten. Once the symptoms just described are evident, there is no cure and the horse should be humanely destroyed.

Care Of The Afflicted Horse

The Sick Stall, Clothing, Feeding, Laxatives, Water, Grooming, Disinfection, Slinging, Restraint.

The Sick Stall

An afflicted horse should be placed in a comfortable box stall that is clean, well bedded down and ventilated, but free of any drafts. Since sick horses often suffer from poor appetite, the atmosphere should be warm if possible to prevent less waste of body tissue. In cases of lameness, sawdust or shavings beddings are preferred over straw, as less depth and bulk enables the horse to move about more easily.

Clothing

If the weather is cold and the stall cannot be artificially heated, the horse should be warmly blanketed. Bandaging the legs loosely with woolen bandages will give additional warmth. If the patient suffers from poor circulation or if the weather is extremely cold, a hood should also be used.

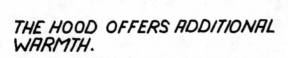

THE HOOD OFFERS ADDITIONAL WARMTH.

Feeding

Some afflicted horses retain a good appetite and care must be taken not to overfeed them. Other horses have impaired appetites and require tempting with special diets. Such cases should be offered bran mashes with rolled oats or honey added. Chopped alfalfa may be dampened with a mixture of molasses and water. Fresh grass, carrots, apples, bread or biscuits are all good foods for tempting a poor appetite. Induce hand feeding if it is necessary, but never force food on a horse. Feed small amounts often and remove any uneaten portions from the feed box.

Laxatives

A lax condition of the bowels, which promotes the excretion of waste, is generally desirable for afflicted horses. Bran mashes have proved satisfactory over the years as mild laxatives and most horses relish them. To make a bran mash, put three to four pounds of bran in a bucket and add enough boiling water to dampen. The thicker the mash, the more readily the horse will eat it. Stir well and cover with a sack for 20 minutes, then feed. Rolled oats may be added to make the mash more palatable. Salt (¾ ounce to the three or four pounds of bran) may also be added.

For a linseed mash, simply make an ordinary bran mash and then add one pint of pure linseed oil. Special precaution should always be taken to use only pure linseed oil. That sold by many merchants, since it is used in painting, has been boiled and mixed with poisons which increase the drying property of the oil.

Epsom salts are also a useful laxative for horses, but their action as a purgative is uncertain. Epsom salts may be given twice a day in doses of four ounces in a bran mash.

Water

A bucket of fresh water should always be kept within easy reach. In extremely cold weather it should be slightly warmed or the chill taken off. Even if the sick horse does not drink, he may frequently wash his mouth out, therefore the water should be changed often.

Grooming

A horse that is very sick should not be unnecessarily groomed. But it is a good practice to sponge out the eyes and nostrils daily, especially if there is any discharge. Hand rubbing the legs is generally beneficial, but anything which upsets the patient should be avoided.

Disinfection

Horses afflicted with any contagious or infectious disease can spread germs of the disease to the surroundings in which they live and to other animals which they come in contact with. Spreading of a disease can be prevented by quarantine and thorough disinfection. A compound creosol solution has proved satisfactory as a disinfectant and Lysol is also recommended. For general stable use, place one tablespoonful of Lysol in one pint of water.

Disinfection, to be successful, requires thoroughness in cleaning and in saturating everything with the disinfecting solution. All stable litter should be burned and the floors flooded with a double strength disinfectant. The stable walls, partitions, mangers, and drinking containers should be scrubbed thoroughly. Any curry combs, brushes, tack, or blankets that came in contact with the diseased horse should also be disinfected. Walls of any buildings, fences, water tanks, and feed boxes in the outdoor pen or corral must not be overlooked.

Slinging

Slings are often used for afflicted horses who are unable to lie down or for resting those who should be kept standing. If used properly, most horses will readily accept the support, but if a sling is not employed properly it can interfere with the animal's breathing and digestion.

The sling should only lightly touch the abdomen when the horse is standing, so that he may rest upon it or not, as he chooses. The sling should be provided with a breastplate and breeching to prevent the horse from slipping forward or back. Be sure the sling is fastened to rafters that are strong enough to support the horse's full weight. Whenever a horse is in a sling he should be checked frequently, day and night.

Restraint

In the management of sick or injured horses special re-

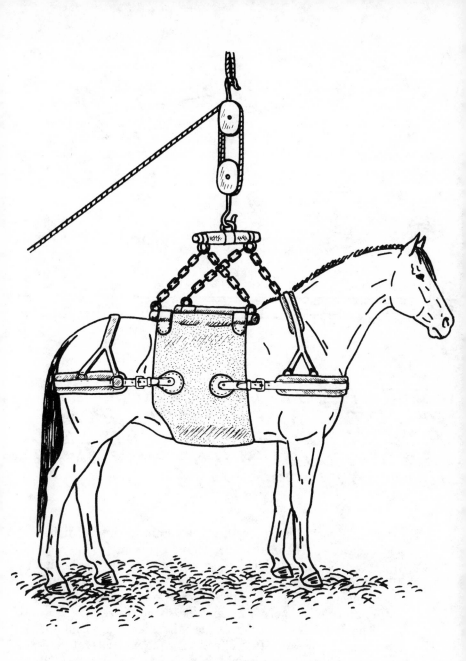

THE SLING IN USE

103

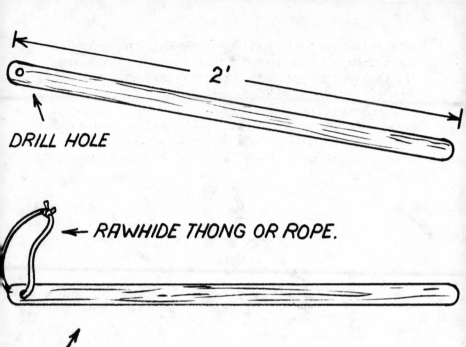

DRILL HOLE

← RAWHIDE THONG OR ROPE.

A TWITCH IS EASILY MADE BY RUNNING A
SMALL PIECE OF ROPE OR RAWHIDE THONG
THROUGH A HOLE IN THE END OF A ROUNDED
PIECE OF WOOD 2 FEET LONG, AND TYING IT
INTO A SMALL LOOP.

straint is sometimes necessary for administering medicines
or medication. The methods vary, and the one to use depends
largely upon the individual horse and the purpose of restraint.
Select only the mildest and least dangerous method. It should
be remembered that kindness, perseverance and tact will
often accomplish more than any means of restraint.

The twitch is one of the simplest, handiest and commonest
methods of restraint. It is effective in the majority of cases,
but it should never be roughly used. The twitch actually shuts

off circulation in the lip and therefore it should never be used continuously over any period of time. To use the twitch, pass the loop over the upper lip (never use on the ears or tongue), which is seized by the left hand and drawn forward. Care must be taken to turn the edges of the lip to prevent injury to the mucous membranes. The cord is then twisted by turning the handle until there is sufficient pressure. When the twitch is removed, rub the lip with the palm of the hand to help restore circulation.

Veterinarian Rectal Thermometer
Syringe for giving medicine internally.
Rubber Syringe for treating wounds
Scissors for clipping hair, removing bandages
Sterile Absorbent Cotton for cleaning wounds, wrapping the legs
Bandages of the cotton surgical type, three to four inches wide
Gauze Pads in two-inch and four-inch squares
Veterinarian Vaseline for use around wounds to prevent hair loss
Boric Acid for washing out the eyes
Epsom Salts for sprains, infection
Tincture of Iodine for use in puncture wounds
Liniment for strains, swelling, inflammation
Antiseptic Dusting Powder for treating open cuts, infected lesions
Thrush Remedy
Analgesic Ointment for chafes, cuts and abrasions
Peroxide of Hydrogen antiseptic for treating wounds
Blood Stop Powder to check capillary bleeding of superficial cuts
Cotton Swabs for removing foreign materials from wounds

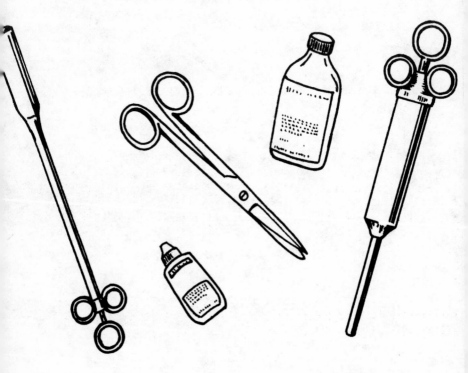

First Aid

Foot Bandage, Puncture Wounds, Deep Wounds, Minor Wounds, Joint Wounds, Proud Flesh, Maggots And Screwworms, Bruises, Leg Bandaging, Sprains, Burns, Eye Injuries, Saddle Sores.

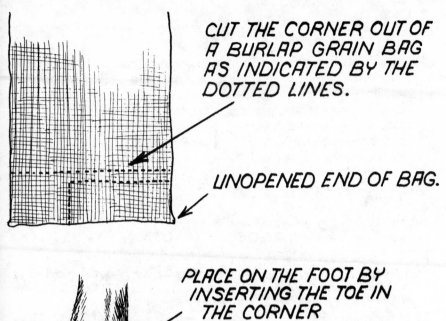

CUT THE CORNER OUT OF A BURLAP GRAIN BAG AS INDICATED BY THE DOTTED LINES.

UNOPENED END OF BAG.

PLACE ON THE FOOT BY INSERTING THE TOE IN THE CORNER

STRIPS

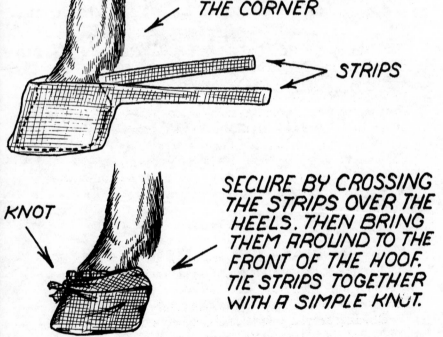

KNOT

SECURE BY CROSSING THE STRIPS OVER THE HEELS. THEN BRING THEM AROUND TO THE FRONT OF THE HOOF. TIE STRIPS TOGETHER WITH A SIMPLE KNOT.

FOOT BANDAGE

Treatment of Wounds

Horses are quite susceptible to wounds from falls, barb-wire fences, nails, splinters, etc. Wounds vary in importance and danger depending on their size and depth. Serious wounds should always be given prompt attention by a veterinarian as suturing and antibiotics may be required. Less serious or minor wounds should be given attention by the horse owner. No wound should ever be considered too minor for treatment. Inflammation, subsequent infection, and even death may arise from the most minor wound if it is untreated.

Puncture Wounds

Puncture wounds are extremely dangerous because the surface generally closes over rapidly and seals back the blood and discharge which should be allowed to escape. Thus a condition is created which breeds tetanus bacteria. Any puncture wound should have the immediate care of a veterinarian, as the administration of tetanus antitoxin and antibiotics are required. If a veterinarian is not immediately available, wash the wound and the area around the wound with warm water and soap. If the opening is small and little bleeding has resulted, it should be aseptically enlarged to remove any foreign material and allow free bleeding. Apply tincture of iodine to the wound with a cotton swab, going in as far as possible. Apply an antibiotic and cover with a bandage. Change the dressing three times daily, syringing out the wound with a mild antiseptic each time. Early administration of tetanus antitoxin is recommended.

Deep Wounds

Deep wounds often bleed profusely and a considerable amount of blood may be lost while you anxiously wait for a veterinarian. Therefore when such emergencies arise, the horse owner should know how to help arrest profuse bleeding.

Bleeding from a vein is easily recognized by the dull red coloring of the blood and its steady, even flow. Copious applications of cold water will generally stop venous bleeding.

In severe arterial bleeding, recognized by the bright scarlet blood which appears in spurts, the wound should be bathed continuously with cold water. If a limb artery has been damaged, a tourniquet may be applied above the wound. The tourniquet, which may be made of a piece of small rope, small rubber tube, or a leather thong, will partly stop the circulation of blood by pressure on the blood vessels. The inexperienced must remember that the tourniquet should not be too tight and it must be loosened at frequent intervals. Destructive changes and eventual death of the part may result if the tourniquet is used for too long a period.

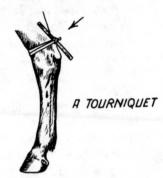

A TOURNIQUET

Once the wound has stopped bleeding, cover it with a clean bandage and keep the horse quiet until the veterinarian arrives.

Minor Wounds

Any bleeding of a wound must be stopped before the wound is treated. Once all bleeding has been stopped carefully clip all hair away from the wound's edges. Then wash the wound thoroughly but gently with warm water. Remove all dirt, clots of blood, and foreign bodies of any kind. Now wash gently with a mild antiseptic. Peroxide of hydrogen is a good antiseptic for cleaning wounds. When dry apply an analgesic ointment which will relieve pain and promote healing. Bandage the wound if possible to keep dirt out. Change the bandage daily and check the condition of the wound. If there is any evidence of discharging pus, the wound must be kept open to maintain drainage. Daily washing with a mild disinfectant and applications of the analgesic ointment must be faithfully carried out until all signs of pus disappear. Once the wound begins to fill in with repair tissue, remove the bandage and leave it off. Long bandaging often prevents wounds from covering themselves with skin and results in the formation of proud flesh.

Any wound near a joint of the leg is considered serious. The development of an "open joint" may result and the loss or infection of the joint fluid often causes permanent stiffness of the limb.

Joint wounds often appear minor at the outset, but within a day or two the joint may begin to swell and gradual stiffness may be noted. As the swelling increases, pain becomes more severe and an oily pus is discharged from the wound. In some cases a fever develops, there is a loss of appetite and the horse is extremely lame, barely touching the floor with the toe of the affected leg.

A veterinarian's services are required for serious joint wounds and in extreme cases the horse may have to be placed in a sling. Minor joint wounds should be thoroughly cleaned and hot applications used. Then the wound may be treated as described for minor wounds.

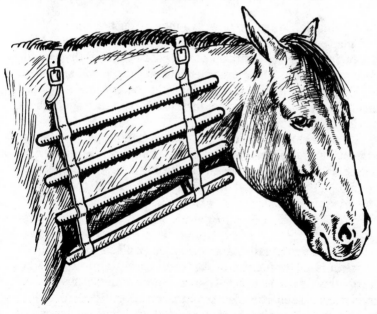

THE CRADLE IS OFTEN USED TO PREVENT HORSES FROM BITING OR LICKING WOUNDS.

Proud Flesh

The presence of proud flesh (excessive granulations) in a wound will prevent or retard healing. It generally occurs in slow healing wounds and is recognized by the rounded fleshy masses which protrude beyond the edges of the wound. It is usually inflamed and ugly looking and bleeds easily. Excessive growth of proud flesh can disfigure or even disable a horse when it is situated near a joint.

Most cases of proud flesh can be prevented by giving all wounds proper care until they are healed. The growth of the fleshy mass may be kept down by removing it with sharp, sterile scissors to the level of the skin, and then treating with tincture of iodine. A bandage applied to exert a mild pressure over the wound has also proved beneficial in some cases. Once developed, proud flesh generally requires surgical removal by a veterinarian.

Maggots and Screwworms

During the warm months wounds often become flyblown and maggots appear. These maggots feed in the horse's skin, producing a severe irritation, and destroy the ability of the skin to function. Their presence is generally recognized by a bloody discharge from the wound and the red, ugly appearance of its edges. If the wound is closely examined, movement of the maggots may be noted.

Remove the visible maggots with sterile forceps or tweezers and then gently swab out the wound with tincture of iodine. If the flies continue to be a problem, the wound should be bandaged or covered with pine tar to repel the flies.

Bruises

Bruises are usually caused by falls or blows and, although the skin is not generally broken, the tissues and muscles beneath the skin are injured. Since the injured tissues become inflamed and sensitive to pressure, lameness often results.

Bruises should never be neglected, as even bruises which

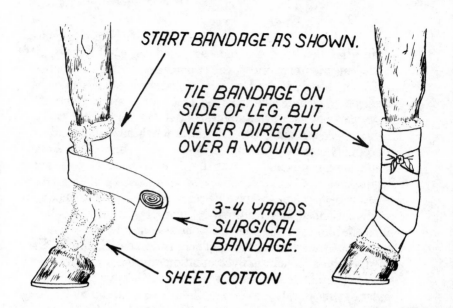

START BANDAGE AS SHOWN.

TIE BANDAGE ON SIDE OF LEG, BUT NEVER DIRECTLY OVER A WOUND.

3-4 YARDS SURGICAL BANDAGE.

SHEET COTTON

NEVER APPLY A WET BANDAGE. IT MAY SHRINK AND PRODUCE SWELLING AND SORENESS.

WHEN COTTON IS USED, BE SURE IT EXTENDS BEYOND THE BANDAGE AT BOTH ENDS.

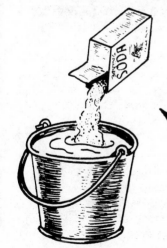

USE FLANNEL BANDAGE FOR COLD WATER TREATMENTS.

ADD COMMON SODA TO WATER TO MAKE WATER COOLER.

LEG BANDAGING

appear minor may become chronic and contribute to serious disabilities involving the muscles, tendons, or the bone.

When it is first noticed, cold compresses should be applied to the bruise. If located on a leg, flannel bandages may be used, but they must be changed frequently, since otherwise they act as hot water bandages. After the cold water treatment, apply a cooling lotion such as witch hazel, and rub it thoroughly around and lightly over the bruise. The horse should be given complete rest until all evidence of pain has disappeared.

If a bruise has escaped notice and the swelling has already developed, hot water or hot compresses should be applied continuously for one or two hours and then at frequent intervals throughout the day. Then a liniment should be applied, rubbing it thoroughly around the edges and lightly over the bruise. Once the swelling, heat, and tenderness have lessened considerably, massage the bruise with liniment once a day for about a week or until all signs of the bruise have disappeared.

Sprains

Muscles, tendons, and ligaments are subject to strain from slips, falls, hard pulling, etc. Sprains may occur anywhere in the horse's body, but they are most frequent in the legs. A full recovery from sprains often takes considerable time and a recurrence of the trouble is quite common.

In cases of mild sprain, cold water applications, followed by massage with a cooling lotion and rest, is all that is normally required. More severe sprains should be bathed with hot water for at least 20 minutes. Dry thoroughly by hand rubbing. When the area is dry, apply a liniment and rub vigorously over the area of the sprain. Repeat this treatment three times a day until swelling and lameness subside. Give the horse complete rest until signs of improvement are evident. Then exercise him mildly, gradually increasing the exercise each day. Severe sprains require the services of a veterinarian, as special bandaging, shoes, blistering, or firing may be required.

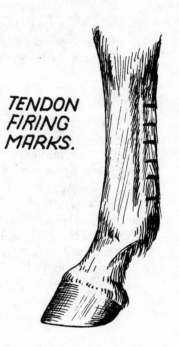

TENDON FIRING MARKS.

Burns

Burns, which may result from a flame, hot solids, steam, liquids, or certain chemicals, are extremely painful and most horses will resent anything but very gentle handling of the affected area.

Minor burns should be treated with a tannic acid jelly, which may be smeared on a sterile gauze pad and then applied to the burn. Follow this with another gauze pad and secure it with a bandage.

In an emergency a strong, warm tea may be used to treat burns. Soak a gauze pad in the warm tea and apply it to the burn. Cover with a dry pad and then bandage.

Baking soda is often used for burns caused by corrosive chemicals. Bathe the burn gently with a solution made by adding one teaspoonful of soda to one pint of warm water.

Extensive burns should be treated by a veterinarian so that suitable narcotics or anaesthetics may be given. Horses suffering extensive burns should be kept warm and offered water, but under no circumstances should water, oil, grease, iodine, or disinfectants be applied to the burn.

Eye Injuries

Eye injuries are generally caused by blows, scratches from wire, or punctures from brush, forage, or nails protruding from mangers, walls, or doorways. They are usually recognized by excessive watering, reddened membranes, a milky coloring, and partial or complete closing of the eye.

Dirt and other small foreign objects are generally removed by carefully flooding the eye with a warm boric acid solution. If the eye was irritated by the foreign matter, repeat the treatment several times a day.

Any serious cut, tear, or puncture of the eye or eyelid should have the immediate attention of a veterinarian.

Saddle Sores

Saddle sores generally result from saddles that do not conform to the shape of the horse's back. As a result there is undue pressure upon the backbone and the flesh is pinched at the sides of the backbone. The repeated irritation will gradually cause a loss of hair and finally a sore.

The best treatment for a saddle sore is complete rest from the saddle until the sore is completely healed. Wash the open sore with a disinfectant and then apply an analgesic ointment daily until healed. The cause of the sore should be corrected before the saddle is used again.

Raw saddle sores may often be avoided if noticed in the early stages of irritation. Apply salt water to the irritated area to harden the skin. Mix three tablespoons of salt to one pint of water. Also promptly correct the condition causing the irritation.

Bibliography

Ensminger, M. E. *Horse Husbandry.* Illinois: Interstate Printers & Publishers, 1951.

A Guide To Lameness & Unsoundness In Horses. New York: Troy Chemical Company, 1952.

Hayes, M. H. *Veterinary Notes For Horse Owners.* New York: Arco Publishing Company, 1970.

Hoof Care. New York: Troy Chemical Company, 1962.

How To Recognize Horse Health Problems. Nebraska: Farnam Horse Library, n.d.

Lyon, W. E. *First Aid Hints For Horse Owners.* London: Collins, 1951.

Miller, Robert E. *Health Problems Of The Horse.* Colorado: The Western Horseman, 1967.

Simmons, Hoyt H. *Horseman's Veterinary Guide.* Colorado: The Western Horseman, 1963.